ALL
THAT
WAS
NOT
HER

CRITICAL GLOBAL HEALTH Evidence, Efficacy, Ethnography
A series edited by Vincanne Adams and João Biehl

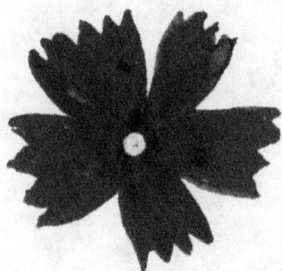

TODD MEYERS

ALL THAT WAS NOT HER

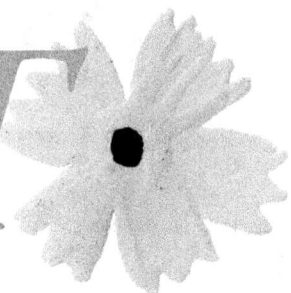

Duke University Press
Durham & London 2022

© 2022 DUKE UNIVERSITY PRESS
DESIGNED BY COURTNEY LEIGH RICHARDSON
TYPESET IN GARAMOND PREMIER PRO
BY COPPERLINE BOOK SERVICES

Cover art: Alma Woodsey Thomas, *Double Cherry
Blossoms*, 1973 (detail). Acrylic on canvas, 60 in. × 40⅛ in.
Courtesy Bowdoin College Museum of Art, Brunswick,
Maine, gift of halley k. harrisburg and Michael Rosenfeld.

Backgrounds and flowers hand-painted
by Allyson Joy Marshall.

Library of Congress Cataloging-in-Publication Data
Names: Meyers, Todd, author.
Title: All that was not her / Todd Meyers.
Other titles: Critical global health.
Description: Durham : Duke University Press, 2022. |
Series: Critical global health |
Includes bibliographical references.
Identifiers: LCCN 2021021966 (print)
LCCN 2021021967 (ebook)
ISBN 9781478015277 (hardcover)
ISBN 9781478017899 (paperback)
ISBN 9781478022510 (ebook)
Subjects: LCSH: Chronic diseases—Maryland—Baltimore—Case studies. |
Chronic diseases —Social aspects —Maryland—Baltimore—Case studies. |
Poor women—Medical care —Maryland—Baltimore—Case studies. |
Medical anthropology —Philosophy. | Chronic diseases —Philosophy.
| Quality of life. | BISAC: SOCIAL SCIENCE / Anthropology /
Cultural & Social | SOCIAL SCIENCE / Sociology / Urban Classification:
LCC RA644.7.M3 M494 2022 (print) |
LCC RA644.7.M3 (ebook) | DDC 616/.044—dc23
LC record available at https://lccn.loc.gov/2021021966
LC ebook record available at https://lccn.loc.gov/2021021967

for Pamela

Undoing

Reassembling

CONTENTS

UNDOING

What follows is an essay about the undoing of an anthropologist who was undone alongside a woman he knew, or tried to know. It is the record of an ending; a test of what one can say or do in the aftermath of an end. She was ill; those around her were ill. He attempted in a small but purposeful way to record the moments in which she unraveled, physically and psychically, and rarer moments when she pulled together. Years passed. The relationship soured. Time is central to this story but not to its length—moments are indiscriminate, shaken from their place along a continuum. Still, it took him a long time to recognize the accumulation of failure. He says this knowing just how phony it must sound. And he may be a phony, but not a modest one. Modesty has no value for the anthropologist, whose discipline requires him to perform virtue and assert truth even while claiming uncertainty and worry. There is certainty here and the wholeness of ruination.

Boo hiss, the final word offers such little satisfaction.

The inventory of minor happenings in the other global South.[1]

A career in the human sciences made in a hollow space.

THESE
MOMENTS
FORMED
BETWEEN
US

I've planned to meet Beverly at her house in the early afternoon. I call to make sure she's home—I'd made the long drive across Baltimore many times before only to be greeted by an unanswered knock at the door or a family member who tells me she's gone elsewhere.

Her son answers the phone and explains that his mother was taken by ambulance to the hospital the night before, after his grandmother found her unconscious on the bathroom floor. He says her condition is bad. He suggests I pick him up so we can go to the hospital together.

I let panic set in.

When we arrive, Beverly's mother is asleep on the bed. Beverly sits in a chair, one arm attached to an IV and the other outstretched, absently picking at food on a cafeteria tray. She's watching the television that hangs high on the wall above her. It takes her a few seconds to notice us before she turns to us and answers a question I'm only thinking: "You should have seen me yesterday." She tells her son to start packing up. Her mother, now awake, staggers into the bathroom and washes her face. Beverly asks, rhetorically, whether I drove.

Within moments we are walking down the hallway. I amble next to Beverly, holding her arm while she holds a catheter bag, some paperwork, bottles and envelopes of medications, and her coat. On the other side, Beverly's son steadies his mother and grandmother, their arms linked. We are a mismatched chain of paper dolls. Beverly's son carries a clear plastic bag containing pajamas, a hospital robe, and uneaten food items. I feel embarrassed and anxious as we fumble toward the exit. I'm uncertain whether Beverly has been discharged from the hospital; I'm uncertain if my arrival was planned by her or just her first opportunity to bolt. I don't ask. Complicit, I am her getaway. I feel duped by the urgency conveyed to me by her son. But mostly I am irritated because I sense that Beverly has taken advantage of me.

We have been here before.

As I drive I turn to Beverly, who sits next to me in the passenger seat, and ask if we can "try not to make this a habit."

Even now I am not exactly sure what I meant, or rather what I hoped to gain; I only know that my irritation had turned to condescension. Looking straight ahead, she says flatly, "This life is a habit. You get used to it."

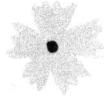

So much of my time with Beverly felt

   repetitive, even mundane, but the monotony

was continually punctured by moments of

      crisis that were hypervolatile.

Life seemed to march steadily on, for better or worse, and then suddenly we were spun around, facing a different horizon. These moments swallowed everyone and everything around Beverly. No one was spared: not me, not her. Crisis would return to her, an awful cycle that brought with it doubt and distrust.

  There was certainly nothing untrue about the crisis that led to her being hospitalized. Later she would tell me about the days of dizziness and clouded thoughts that culminated in her collapse. But the tentacles of falsehood grew from it all the same, ensnarling and smothering its truth. Hospital staff would come to regard her as a pariah. Her son would make apologies. I would lose faith. She would weather their scrutiny and mine. These were little moments of injury, strung together; events that seemed to lay traps for thinking, moments that made it hard to find the right register for apprehending the force of what was happening to her. Or worse, these little moments invited misinterpretation, burying their corrosiveness in misunderstanding; moments that created an opening for some false lesson to be made from this woman.

The following chapters are a record of these moments, of their withering force; an essay about the consuming power of these moments written by a young white anthropologist who followed a middle-aged Black woman and her family for years. In his writing, this younger man now meets his older self at a different political moment, looking back through a distorted lens. Return, here, is itself an action of change, a deformation, and an acknowledgment of that change. I return to write about illness and other injuries not to explain them but to unthread them, or better still, to unravel clues about how they came to be lived as they were lived, how they entangled Beverly and me.

I am also engaged in another kind of unthreading. I direct this essay against a galling, late liberal project that would maintain a set of abstract principles about how things are or how one should be in relation to others—a project that at its core wrongly assumes all forms of living are somehow already known or played out. I refuse to rob living of its terrible inventiveness. If anthropology arranges its politics to counter narratives that demean and vilify, then in equal measure anthropology should admit the danger of cheap moralisms. By unthreading moments, I am looking for something in my encounters with Beverly that is difficult to name. I focus on small, intimate moments of contact and abrasion that offer, at least for me, a way to open and move within a critique of power that flows between two people in order to show, as Elizabeth A. Povinelli suggests, how "the critique of power might impact at a deeper, richer level with immanent forms of social obligation beyond given articulations of identity."[1] By returning to these moments between us—moments that are fine and dense and largely insignificant in some larger scheme—I hope to show what the terms of social obligation expose in their unmaking, expressed by the lack of givenness between Beverly and me.

Beverly and me.

"How does one inhabit these more awkward

worlds of obligation and analyze the differentials

of power shooting through them?"[2]

Indeed. Gone is my sense of how things are meant to go. I had no idea what shape this inquiry would take as it took shape, and even now, its form—in the text and in the reception of the text—is uncertain. This is not a problem of authorship in pursuit of objectivity or the generalization of knowledge; rather it is the epistemological character of arranging words and events with feltness and memory. My challenge, as an actor and author, has been to track this arrangement, wherever it leads.

The minutes and hours we were together, the textual record of that time in my notes, and the faulty memory that wishes to transform touch and old words into new words on the page cannot be taken for granted— two people who were different in so many ways, two people who shared something between them, who inexplicably returned to each other again and again. She entered the relationship differently than I, and she would surely see me differently now. I entered, too, but in order to take her in, to see her, as Stephen Best writes, I had "to enter through a different door."[3]

Beverly's life was a habit. I followed her, habitually. I do not have to guess where the power to think *habitually*—to take up residence in another's life and to repeat that action of habitation over and over, to possess the power to leave or stop or to take an altogether different path— comes from. I also do not have to guess from where the constraint Beverly felt derives. It is a power generated by race and infinite strata of differences and inequalities, "rooted in the material conditions in which those inequities thrive."[4] It strikes me now that in all my years of following Beverly through medical environments, my access was never questioned, not once. I belonged. It strikes me now how many times I watched as security guards asked Beverly to show them the contents of her bag or chided her for being late or early. She belonged to these places, not to possess but to be possessed; she needed, and that need constrained her and was exploited by others.

Beverly knew the scrutiny of others. But Beverly invited me in again and again, to bear the intimacy of scrutiny.[5] It is impossible for me not to think of Beverly when reading the following passage from Audre Lorde: "As we learn the intimacy of scrutiny and to flourish within it, as we learn to use the products of that scrutiny for power within our living, those fears which rule our lives and form our silences begin to lose their control over us."[6] Despite injury and insult, Beverly found a form in which to flourish, knowing only too well the intimacy of scrutiny. I witnessed the unharmonious and threatening reality of this flourishing, and my effort to record and engage it feels both weak and necessary. Her effort to communicate and direct my record feels both tenuous and vital. Christina Sharpe describes this vitality-in-being in a way that drains it of any passivity: "Black being that continually exceeds all of the violence directed at Black life; Black being that exceeds that force."[7] My account is a pale record of this violence and what launches from it. I grab at small bits of its evidence whizzing past in the tempest of that wild and deliberate force, in one life.[8]

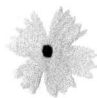

In the case of a life.

The case is a distillation not of many worlds but of a world: the case breaks the smooth tension on the surface of a world seen from above; it is a method of agitating as much as looking, diving in where one sees no bottom.[9] The question of the individual, situated in time but out of step with its familiar cadence; a subject at once the center of clinical and experimental knowledge and pushed to a margin by the mess of living—these are aspects of the intellectual labor of ethnography. My concern with a life, one marked by the real threat of persistent, unrelenting chronic illness, is bounded by the reality of precarity and harm that derive from racism and other prejudices found in the everyday of the world in which Beverly lives. There is nothing neutral in looking back at these moments. What I seek to avoid is "looking through a racially impervious lens" that would ignore the shape of these inequities; at the same time, I seek to avoid conjuring racial tropes.[10] I seek to write the negative without vandalizing it. So clear in our present political moment is how easily racialized fantasies work their way into the representation of Black lives, even or especially in the face of so much struggle.[11] There are failures in the project of late liberalism that we must get into; we must find ways into their unease and contaminating mess. My approach is to use an intimate and frank register to examine those failures, to consider the way they take up residence in lives and how we might exceed them. I ignore the empty promise of an ethics of encounter that is already worked out in advance, removed from Beverly, yet would seek to explain her. The essay risks itself in order to open such a critique. I rely warily on difference; I move within it in order to thwart, as Audre Lorde puts it, a "total denial of the creative function of difference" that would prevent us from saying something, anything, of consequence.[12]

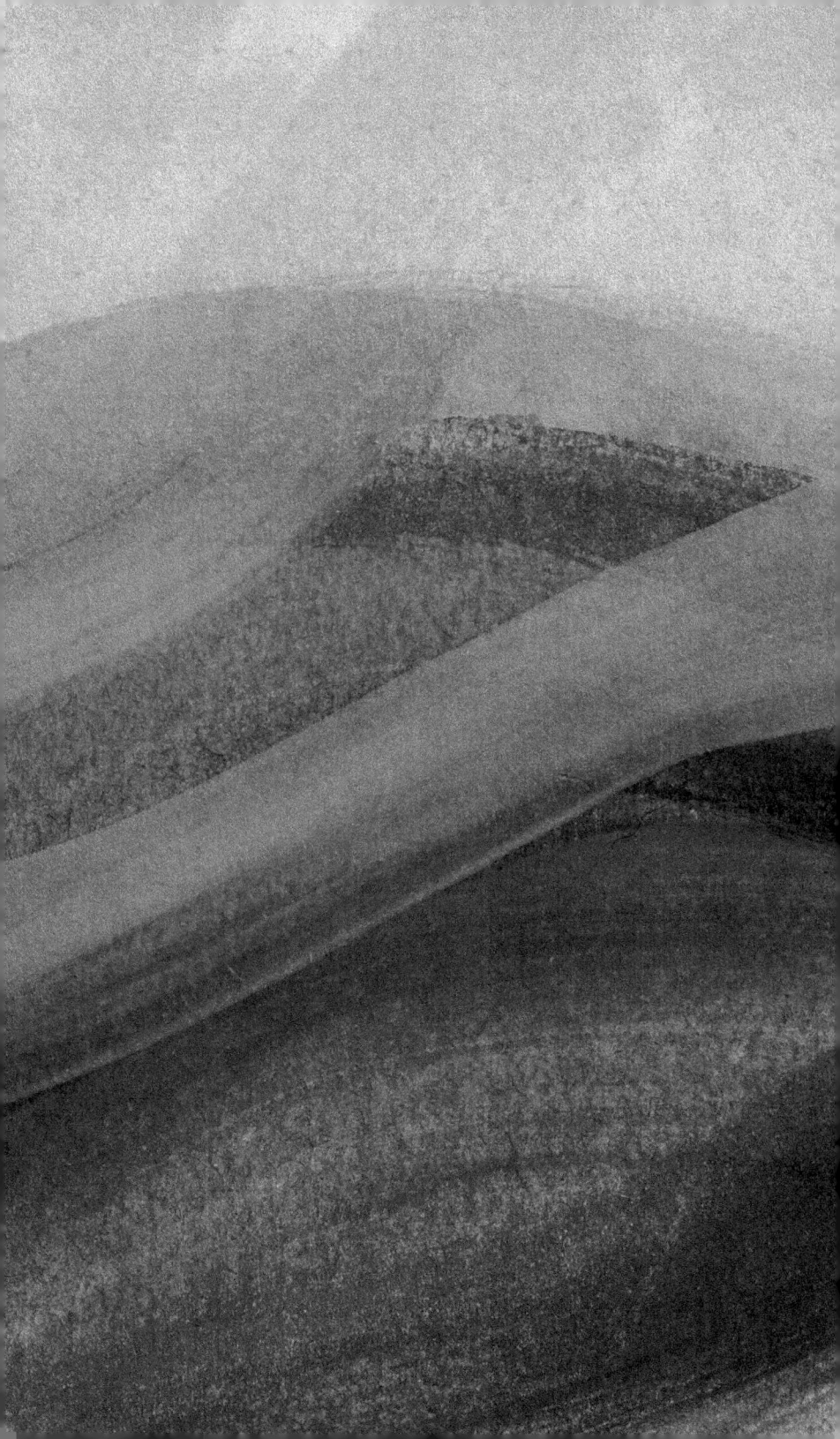

She was there whole, looking exactly as she had at the beginning, capable of the same actions and no more, having the same name, the same habits, the same history. Yet, freed from the block, the relations between her and everything which was not her had changed. An absolute yet invisible change. She was now at the center of what surrounded her. All that was not her made space for her.

JOHN BERGER, *Bento's Sketchbook*

2

STILL
LIFE

For more than a decade he assembled and disassembled the image of a woman, in hospitals and clinics, in the offices of social workers and counselors, in her home. One image became many. Some images deteriorated over time; others were erased. A few sit dormant, untouched. He also gathered images of the things that surrounded this woman, her objects and ether. In her living room, sitting for hours, words like dust on rays of sunshine gone between swirling contrails of cigarette smoke as Beverly passed through the room—her room of nutty, disinfected air, of lavender or pine mixed with the perfume of cooking oil and strong soap. So much of his time in Beverly's living room went unrecorded, or at most was reduced to one or two lines in his notebook after what felt like empty days of fieldwork. Nothing but clutter contained by walls of peeling wallpaper and matted shag carpet, and yet her living room was a place that could crush you. He had been crushed there, in her room, a place she laid claim to, trapped for hours, staring out an open window across the street to an adjacent parking lot at dusk, the miasma of cool air converging with fast food and cut grass. There was no event, no consequence, just the dim purgatory of that room before he climbed back into his car to drive across Baltimore to his home.

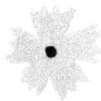

Between moments of nothingness

　　(middleness, in-betweenness) he has been writing

the image of Beverly's body.

The body of an African American woman struggling with chronic illness, wheezing and coughing, a pincushion of diabetes lancets and syringes, on a couch, immobile, then on the move from place to place in the passenger seat of his car or next to him on a bus, making their way to a clinic appointment. A body of aggressive presence, and then, after a period of estrangement, vanished from his sight. Hers was a body held together as much by medical intervention as by memory and loss, now held in his writing, suspended between the fluid action of repair and the final product of a reconstruction.

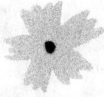

He sits with a sketchbook filled with a collection

of images, drawings in words and figures,

> *some incomplete and others just a few scratches*

on the page, with many years between the time

> > *he made those initial marks and now.*

As he revisits these lines, he wishes he had made them a little sharper in the moments during or soon after shapes were revealed. He finds himself shading forms from memory, in the absence of a subject, from a constellation of hints and errant strokes: the incomplete labor of *Homo depictor*.[1] He finds himself dismantling images, deciphering through repetition and refinement, pursuing forms that felt more complete before his words touched them, forms that would just as soon be left alone.

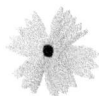

He has become resentful of writing

that begins with conclusions. This is both

his confession and a thesis statement.

He is bitter about words that speak uncertainty in the language of certitude. He winces at every neologism. He is not complaining about the conventions of writing or even the habits of thought that help words attach themselves to things found in the world; he is talking about the danger of ethnography as a sham crucible. Beverly impeded the easy translation of the scene to the word. Over time his vocabulary shrank. He would retreat into titanic signifiers like *illness* and *health* and *care*, words not so much drained of meaning as steadily emptied of his comprehension. Despite being quite ill—and those around her being ill as well—Beverly pulled him away from his preoccupation with chronic illness, or rather caused him to lose confidence in the kind of attention illness demands. But chronic illness remains the through line of this story whether he likes it or not.

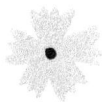

He went searching for Beverly in the

images that surrounded her.

He returned to one image, a picture that exposed how a moment of coming apart took place, a scene where a photographic portrait is central to an event, a scene that exposes the labor undertaken by this portrait in a moment of crisis. It is a scene that shows how the image might be turned fibrous as it weaves time and place, across different scales of anthropological sites (a body, a home, a family, an action, a record of these things in writing, a line, a thread—the unraveled thread being another sort of line). Said plainly, this image offers a way to think through a moment in Beverly's life that enfolds presence—many moments out of time that come into the present well after the fact.

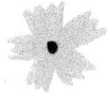

Some things are clear.

A young girl, Beverly's niece, her sister's daughter, is taken from the home in the midafternoon. Or she simply leaves. The family is devastated. He receives a call. When he arrives, the situation has worsened from the one described by Beverly's son on the phone. He asks whether anyone has called the police. He insists that they call, but they do not.

Some things are less clear. He is told that a group of men took the girl. No one recognized them. The men said nothing. There was no struggle. The family does not know why she was taken. Later, when pressed, the authors of these stories will amend what they had said earlier or abandon their versions of events entirely. By the time he arrives at Beverly's house, the girl's mother has placed a photograph of her daughter on a shelf above the television. It's a middle school graduation photo; the girl is smiling as she looks back across her shoulder at the camera; her graduation gown is bright-red satin. Tea candles surround the framed photograph; plastic flowers have been placed on either side, a small bowl of perfumed potpourri at the center.

Beverly's sister is in the bathtub, sobbing. Beverly's youngest son asks him to help lift his aunt out of the tub. He braces himself, anticipating the embarrassment of seeing her naked, but they find her soaking with her clothes on. The house is filled with her ache.

Perhaps the photograph aids contemplation as the family keeps watch, waiting for a phone call, hoping she'll walk back through the door. Beverly tells him she has asked for a miracle. She prays for the girl to be returned. He asks why they are not at the girl's mother's house instead of Beverly's, and her son tells him they want to be close to the place from where she was taken, which contradicts what he was told over the phone about the site of the abduction (his word, *abduction*). He questions nothing. The photograph will remain on the shelf until she returns. And when she does, her mother takes it down and throws it in the garbage. The cheap gilded frame is broken, and the photograph is creased under the glass.

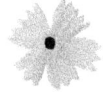

He replays these moments

over and over in his mind.

He drives to Beverly's house. The girl's mother is sobbing. They carry her to the bedroom, place her on the bed, and dry her with towels and a blanket. He goes downstairs. He says he is willing to call the police. "Won't do no good," Beverly tells him. He says they can give names, some people her niece knows, friends. Or maybe they can call hospitals. He insists. Beverly at first ignores him and then cuts him off. She tells him if he calls the police, she won't tell them anything.

"Tell them what? What will you tell them?" she asks angrily.

She turns cold.

She tells him if he calls the police, the girl's mother will tell them he had something to do with her going missing. She says, "We'll tell them you did something."

He barely responds; he is not even sure if he did. The air is sucked from his lungs. He leaves without a word. He returns to his car. He sits, slumped. He is too shocked to drive, so he sits there—fearful, stupid, impotent.

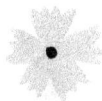

Days later she calls.

He braces himself and returns.

The niece came home in the middle of the night. Or was returned. The photograph is now in the kitchen garbage; the small objects that surrounded it are still on the shelf. The smells of body odor and sex and food being prepared hang in the air. The niece is on the couch, staring blankly, sucking her thumb. The aunt sits in the kitchen, her face ashen.

He has no words for Beverly. He cannot tell if she's gloating or about to cry, or scream. He notices she has dug her fingernails into the palms of her hand, dashes of Morse code in dried blood.

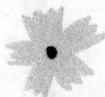

What use is it to return to this scene, to engage

in the unpleasant and intrusive task of pushing up

against images that resist revealing themselves,

images that are in fact hostile to knowing?

He pores over these images again. They do not hold still. He says he is sorting out their meaning, but in truth he feels desperate to attach meaning to them. Something sent him back "to rethink scenes over and over again," maybe to move closer than he had before, maybe to mend them in some way.[2]

There is also something about repeating scenes in writing—captioning these moments as an act of protection that, through their repetition, somehow insulates him from them. Beverly's sister's relation to the middle school photograph was devotional, certainly, but as an image it did something else as well. Something was pressed up against it and then released. Maybe it was her child as a child in a moment of an eclipsing childhood. Was there guilt? In her grief, did he detect complicity? Then as now he has no confidence in his understanding. He has his own thoughts and suspicions, seeds of resentment that are hard to unsow. If he had called the police, would the girl have been murdered? What could he have said knowing next to nothing? Was she taken or given away? Or maybe these readings fail to apprehend the event altogether. The photograph forced something to change and, in a moment of transformation, was discarded. Perhaps it had to be discarded because, to use John Berger's words, it held a "thereness . . . that refuses moderation or self-protection."[3] The photograph is an image that sat there on the shelf and sits there in the pit of his stomach still.

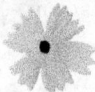

Careers are made through the trope of suffering,

told through stories that reflect the celebrity

and intrepidness of their authors, stories that

refract the image of another's unraveling.

He offered so little. Car rides. On occasion he could share information about health services; he helped to fill out benefits and insurance claims forms. He would occasionally buy meals. He listened. He offered attention and sympathy at times when the odds were against this woman. She always seemed to pull through, but nothing was ever guaranteed. She endured things that would end others, he is certain. She was sick. But she managed illness after illness, symptom after symptom, a web of symptoms that made her, to use her phrase, "one sick lady." But that was not all. She cared for others; she absorbed crisis after crisis, and these were woven between the lattices of her sickness like ribbons. In his attempts to recount these moments with her, these ribbons were pulled out and discarded for reasons that were never clear, making new shapes and patterns but never changing fully the thing that held them. Beverly remained. The pattern of her only appeared different at different times.

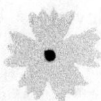

Dreadful, but look on the bright side.

He finds the contest between the anthropology of hope and the anthropology of suffering tedious. Beverly is not a product of a disciplinary dispute premised on competing humanisms. But how to show the ways hope and despair—only two shades among hundreds of other gradations—modulate life, outline and distort life in the same stroke? How to inscribe a life with a line?

Berger describes drawing from the point of contact between the instrument and the paper. The hand makes an assessment of the paper's absorbency, its smoothness, the give or resistance, and then modifying pressure, tests and retests, again and again, how best to make one mark and then the next.[4] Perhaps writing and rewriting these scenes, redrawing them, is a way to test the instrument while thinking what form that instrument is attempting to secure—to resemble a form as he sees it, or saw it, which blends his perspective and the one Beverly offered him, hoping never to confuse the two. But none of this feels satisfying, let alone a creative act. It is the art of dismantling facts and near facts to divulge a form that is already there, observable but surrounded by a substance dense with factness and emotion and regret. Beverly and he worked through images, formed and deformed a mosaic of images (of illness, of care, of their relationship, of other things as well), moments and words that imprinted themselves as images, tiny pieces that fit together unevenly. The portrait, the girl's disappearance, her return, the recriminations that followed, and his doubts about the circumstances surrounding her vanishing made a new, untamable image, heavy and opaque and savage—an image filled with other images that surrounded the portrait (a young woman sucking her thumb, her mother's moans heard from the porch before he stepped into the house, her mother slamming dishes into the kitchen sink while her daughter watched television vacantly from the couch).

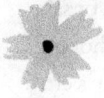

He has abandoned any attempt to reduce these years to a few meager pages.

Such thinking only amplifies what little these pages can do. The page is a weak scaffold upon which the things of a life are held, and to be sure, this work knows its author's weakness—weakness, not always failure, but something diminished. As a medical anthropologist he straddles disciplines that either see the virtue in health as a given or see the terms of that virtue as continually in need of testing. His erosion of confidence in this entire enterprise results from his subject's power to erode. If there is a point, it is to say things convincingly, because to be sure, in this tell-ing, even breathing feels like a falsehood. This is his attempt to word the image, to return texture to it, to rewet a faded gouache.

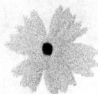

The tension of health and illness is inseparable from other tensions, other conflicts and joys visited upon Beverly and her family.

And then there were things that were horrible, real horrors. A girl taken, the shock of her family's response, their cruelty and self-interest—stability, coherence, none of this returns, and even when she returned, she really didn't. Long hours of nothing, the something-nothing of anthropology, then the dizzying punctuation of crisis, its awfulness, the specter of an assault, and even in the midst of it all there is the impulse to forget, to wish it away, to remain aloof. Maybe we can call this tendency the failing ethics of the encounter, but he prefers to think with these moments not because they are unethical or horrible, but precisely because they offer an ethics that has yet to be worked out. Encounters take hold; they get under the skin and get stuck in the image of thought, unrelenting, and for the anthropologist who hopes to write about these encounters, they dare us to betray their truth, to acknowledge their dim force.

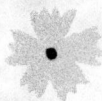

How carefully must we approach the image

in words, to unflatten the experience of illness

and harm through language, when life seems to

happen somewhere off to the side of language?[5]

Susan Stewart offers clues when she describes the trap laid by language in the painting of a still life, warning that "language gives form to our experience, providing through narrative a sense of closure and providing through abstraction an illusion of transcendence."[6] The still life instead dwells; it transcends nothing. And like Giorgio Morandi, who painted hundreds of *nature morte* of bowls and other ceramics with the same or similar compositions, the artist of the still life does not freeze the image but simply lingers with it for an extended period, departs, and returns to a different image of the same. Perhaps that is where value is found. Persistence. Nearness. Return. Reinvention. Others have described it in different ways.[7] This is the contact of the instrument and paper. Beverly takes shape as an image in his ethnography, between objects and other forms, as the product of affects and misinterpretations and intimacies that are out of step with what seems good and right, what so easily—so expectantly—calls out for the single, flattened image of her.

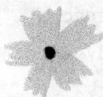

The image is a photograph, a middle school graduation portrait of a girl, chin down, head tilted, wide smile, hair freshly straightened, crimson cap and gown; a gold tassel more yellow than the gilded frame that holds the photograph brushes her cheek.

The photograph sits atop a large television, surrounded by tea candles, with potpourri in the center, plastic flowers on either side. The portrait is a nothing that has become a something in the wake of an event. The portrait cannot melt back into the chorus of cousins and other relatives lining the walls and shelves of Beverly's living room, to rejoin them, insignificant and unbroken. The girl's mother placed the photograph on the television after the girl ran away or was taken. It would never return.

That was what he saw, what he was told, and all he would come to know. There was just enough conveyed over the telephone to get him in his car and to the house presumably to help in whatever way he could. Little splinters of the scene had been pulled off and pressed back together to complete the image of an event.

The portrait was of a child at a moment that marked a future, her expression filled with pride. When her mother placed the image on the television, it was dropped like an anchor in time, hitched to some point before the disappearance of this girl now unmoored. And it was an image that could no longer be tolerated upon her eventual return because it trespassed on her real presence in the living room after days of absence. She departed and then returned, and the portrait was no longer welcomed. She, her presence, forced a choice about who would remain and who would not. Now she sat cross-legged on the couch, hair teased out clumsily to one side, body odor hanging in the air, sucking her thumb, her face void. She was there and far off. She was now at the center of what surrounded her. All that was not her made space for her.

The time is gone when mere accidents could still happen to me; and what could still come to me now that was not mine already? What returns, what finally comes home to me, is my own self and what of myself has long been in strange lands and scattered among all things and accidents.

FRIEDRICH NIETZSCHE, "The Wanderer," from *Thus Spoke Zarathustra*

3

THE
ACCIDENT
OF
CONTACT

I know less about Beverly now than when I met her nearly two decades ago. When the relationship began, I had very little idea where it would lead. At the time, I wanted to know how families living in situations of serious economic and social insecurity, in situations of deep uncertainty, in the context of racial prejudice and exception, came together to meet the challenges of caring for someone with chronic illness, of *together* coping with chronic illness. I am still interested in this question, perhaps more concerned than interested, as things have arguably worsened for families in Baltimore. I continued to talk with one family, one woman in this family, for years after our first meeting. The scope of that conversation, of what it was that I was doing as an anthropologist through a relationship that was different than friendship—a relationship that splintered over and over—evolved in ways that make it hard to see all the changes in course along the way.

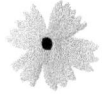

She shared so much of her from the

beginning, and there was so much

of her left unaccounted after the end.

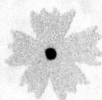

I met Beverly through colleagues while
she was fulfilling community service hours
　　　　by answering phones at a public-housing
rental office after a minor drug offense.

She had agreed to be one of thirty families enrolled in a study aimed at better understanding how illness is managed in low-income households. After I had made a few visits to her home, she asked if we could continue meeting.

Maybe the anticipation of an audience was one reason she spoke with me, or continued to speak with me. She wanted to be heard. There were times the audience seemed to widen beyond the two of us as she spoke, giving her speech the tone of a sermon. Other times, every utterance felt like we had made a secret pact.

But why this beginning and not another? What was formed by the accident of contact that made returning over and over possible—what was the quality of that encounter? In all my years of field notes I find no evidence of this moment, a scribble on the back of my hand smudged into extinction long ago. There is nothing I have found in my notes that counts as a moment of adhesion. I was overeager and took the absurdity of our connection for granted; I failed to acknowledge all the unevenness between us. Now, in this moment, in a different moment, I so desperately want to tell the story differently—how I met Beverly, how I slowly built rapport and cultivated a relationship—but there is no story to tell. Even in my own accounting I come into the picture of us much later, when things begin to come apart.

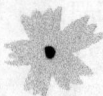

I focused on her ailments.

Arthritis
       Migraines
             "Dizziness"
        Chronic Obstructive Pulmonary Disease
"Confusion"
           Depression
               Substance Abuse
                  Type 2 Diabetes Mellitus

Hypertension

Hepatitis C

Obesity

Kidney Disease

"Voices"

Chronic Pain

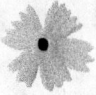

I took crooked inventory.

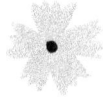

I found list making easy.

It had a purposefulness that answered the question of what it was I was up to even when I failed to grasp what it was I was up to. Honestly, what was I doing anyway, besides prying? Was I working out the scale of how bad things were or would likely become for this woman? I told myself these cross-examinations would lead to something, some action of aid. In the moment, many moments that were repeated again and again, I tried to piece together the whole of a person who I thought had been split apart in the faulty situations of care in which she found herself. She was many kinds of patients, many Beverlys, scattered across different medical environments; in her house, she was caregiver and was cared for, frail and fierce. I was attempting to unify these scattered pieces, these hers, to return them to a single whole that could tolerate the many. My effort may have been exhaustive—it was certainly exhausting and very likely annoying from Beverly's point of view—but in the end there was no wholeness, no repair, no collection of diagnoses to complete a picture—a picture for whom? There were so many pieces, loose pieces of her churning in a sea of other pieces, with a significance that would bob in and out of view.

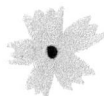

I now harvest little details of her

　　　　　　　　　　　that feel prosaic and unkind.

I remember her skin on that first day, how it was dull brown and dusty with eczema. Her lips were dry, and when she smiled, the deep-yellow ocher of nicotine between her teeth gave the appearance of massive gaps. She smiled and laughed; we laughed. God only knows about what. Maybe laughter was the connective tissue between us, as improbable as it seems. For our first interview I arrived on her doorstep dressed in a white collared shirt, slacks, and a sport jacket. When she invited me in, she told me I looked like a Jehovah's Witness, and I asked if she had accepted Jesus Christ as her Lord and Savior.

Laughter.

She wore a long cotton T-shirt, probably a pajama top that was made to look like an athletic jersey, the neck stretched out, baggy and ill fitting. Printed on the T-shirt was the number 33. I don't know why, but I told her that the number 33 was under the label of every bottle of Rolling Rock beer, how competing mythologies had grown around its meaning that included everything from Freemasonry to devil worship. She said, "You're talking, but all I hear is 'beer.'"

Laughter.

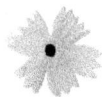

We deserved each other, she and I,

in the worst possible way.

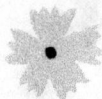

She carried a weight

I could hardly apprehend.

She was so powerful, so compelling and complex, so feeble and elusive, and I knew how easy it would be to garble what I saw and felt of her, to allow our moments together to gelatinize through my writing into prejudice.

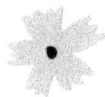

After those first few encounters,

I thought about her all the time.

Even my worry and frustration at a distance felt productive; it felt like I touched her, I remained touching her.

At first there was a sport to our meetings, when they happened, which they often did not. We would play cat and mouse. Unreturned phone calls and unanswered doorbells would take a dramatic turn into panicked answering-machine messages and demands for me to drop everything and visit her. Silence made the way for seemingly endless speech filled with urgency, real urgency. Every encounter had a double in an avoided encounter, but when we met and spoke, there was an intensity that suggested importance. I wanted these moments to be important, to last. *I wanted.* It felt important, this contact. *Our contact.* And her intensity endured well beyond these moments of contact.

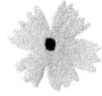

Beverly is now the sour smoke

of spent firecrackers, staining my fingers

and filling my nostrils.

She coats my throat, the thick film of contact that lingers. *Lingering, adamant, in things adjacent to her*. Hers was the heavy perfume of laundry detergent and mothballs that saturated her clothes and her house, a perfume I carried home with me, that eventually worked its way into my car upholstery and my home. I also carried with me the aroma of fry grease, of cigarette smoke, dizzying confusion, anger, and boredom. I carried back and forth the paper record of images I clung to and now question. I wonder if I clung to her as she clung to me, to the things of her, each time I left.

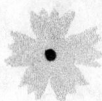

I cling still.

In our encounters we returned to moments in her life again and again. The repetition was reinforcing, not always the facts contained in those exchanges, but the fact that the exchanges were in fact happening at all: the arrogant certainty that they would happen again. When she shared her life, my tentacles grew into her, into her past, making me feel indispensable to the idea of her past, to our work of memory, or so I thought. At times she called our conversations "helping with memory"; other times she called it "scouring shit." In both cases we returned to her past again and again, scouring, together.

I want to return to those moments of shared thought, to the moments when I made these records of her past, now so far out of reach. My memory, even my notes, has little access to the person she was and whom I hoped to preserve. I am the nameless narrator of W. G. Sebald's *The Rings of Saturn*, faced with the distorting distance of time between my thoughts in the now and a thing once admired and misunderstood then: "At the time I could no more believe my eyes than I can now trust my memory."[1]

Beverly is less legible to me now because all the hopes and dreams and delusions and callousness and beauty she shared with me resist retelling from the place I began. That place is gone. My tendency has been to write out of the precarity of Beverly's life, something that has failed me so far as I try to account for her ability to move within her own story, has failed to help me appreciate her movement from someone who performed daily struggles to a companion in the imaginings of her world. To bring her into view now is to accept that the moments of her life to which I bore some witness do not fill out a larger picture, do not help to complete her, and cannot return her to the place where I had once recorded them. These moments are only faintly aware of each other. I suppose the form a portrait takes is nothing more than pale contact between these moments anyway, a halo of sour smoke that gives little shape to her.

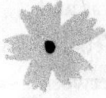

The faintness of her, her color and her voice, has not left me.

I know I am the wrong person for the job, then as now, to do the work of remembrance through a stain.

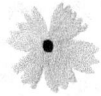

We met.

We are meeting here again. I return to her through imperfect contact. Still, there are different moments in this story, different tenses that refuse to be elided in the final telling. What can I repair of this time? I failed to understand so much of what she offered me. How can I account for our beginnings, to say with confidence that the version of this woman, here, is the version I had vowed to tell? How to return what was taken? Or, as John Berger asks, "Is it possible to send promises backwards?"[2]

Time arrested, as the triumph of metaphor, or so it would seem at first. Perhaps, though, it's more a crisscrossing and slippage of emotion, which you can only recount through descriptions which serve the dead and the living indiscriminately.

DENISE RILEY, *Time Lived, without Its Flow*

4

RESUSCITATIONS

Beverly is gone, but some things remain.

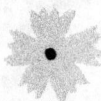

There is a fable he tells himself.

It is a story about a person who experiences physical death but remains a living, breathing subject in the writing and thought of the anthropologist, even when that subject, strictly speaking, no longer lives or breathes. It is the morbid trick of anthropology, to traffic between life and death through scholarly acts of resuscitation, planting the subject in an afterlife where they can be returned to again and again.

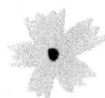

Afterlife.

Beverly's afterlife is really afterlives, two subjects—two Beverlys—equally fierce and unyielding in their insistence on holding forth, asserting themselves in present time, struggling to direct the meaning and force of that presence, pushing through an onslaught of symptoms, balancing family obligations, and negotiating physical limitations. There is the Beverly he holds in the presence of writing, sustained by the productive fiction of anthropological thought in his scholarly life—an unwitting fiction that helps him think through the arbitration of health and illness in situations of social and economic insecurity; the tale of a woman forever on the brink of catastrophe and death, from which she would pull back again and again. And then there was the Beverly who stayed in Baltimore after he left—who died there, a loss to which he was oblivious.

His dilemma has been to sort out these simultaneous Beverlys, both present and absent, insistent about remaining fully in the ledger of Beverly's many episodes of illness (in his notes and through her family's recollections), the record or container through which the movement of time is itemized.[1] Neither Beverly is willing to depart.

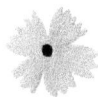

When he thinks of Beverly, he thinks of

   Carrie Mae Weems's Kitchen Table Series *(1990),*

twenty photographs of a Black woman sitting at

   her kitchen table under a bright dining-room light,

each photograph staged, so carefully composed, yet

still retaining something raw, something authentically

domestic and otherwise unobserved or overlooked.

Subtle changes to the background and a revolving cast of actors who feature in one or two photographs give a sense of movement through time, of forward motion. He knows for so long he misunderstood Weems's photographs, or, better, misrecognized Beverly's image in them. The photographs are not windows into the household through the kitchen. They are not snapshots to be looked back upon from some future point in time. He now sees the woman in these photographs as forever held in place, at the table. As others pass freely in and out of the kitchen, she remains. She is held there, returned to, endlessly.

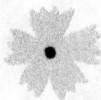

When he left, she told him that

he was always welcome to return.

At the time, it was something he never intended to do.

He stood outside her door, knocking for several minutes, knowing that an unanswered knock did not necessarily mean that no one was home. (How many times had he stood there knocking?) As he felt himself giving up, he saw one of her neighbors crossing the street, and he asked whether she had seen Beverly. "Oh, no, hon, she died a few years ago," the woman said in long, sympathetic tones offered in a Baltimore accent with which he was so familiar. "I'm sorry. But her kids live round here somewhere."

By chance he found her eldest grandson a few doors down from where Beverly once lived. He knew it was Thomas instantly. From the sidewalk several feet below the porch, he could see the top of her grandson's head as he struggled to open the door from his wheelchair. He explained that he knew his grandmother, and that they had met years ago. Her grandson showed no surprise as he invited him in: "I remember you brought us kid books." Her grandson told him he always seemed to be around.

The layout of the row house mirrored Beverly's former home. Whereas Beverly's house had been stiflingly cluttered, her grandson's house was nearly empty; a coffee table was all that sat in the living room, an overfilled ashtray as its centerpiece. Beverly's house had shrunk over the years he knew her. When she was unable to move up and down the stairs, a cot appeared in her living room, allowing her to stay downstairs. Her closet was emptied onto a small table at the end of the sofa; her collection of shoes was arranged along the floor in front of the sofa so that when he sat down he either had to stretch his legs over them or rest his shoes on the pair immediately below where he sat. When her mother stayed with her, a reclining chair and the area around it transformed into a small bedroom complete with nightstand and makeup mirror. When Beverly would regain some semblance of health, these changes would remain—and with each episode of illness, the room would shrink a little more.

Thomas lived with his younger brother. Their sister lived farther down the block with her infant daughter. The only evidence that two young men occupied this house was the autographed Baltimore Ravens football jersey that hung crookedly on the wall of the foyer. Thomas apologized for the absence of chairs in the living room: "I only need the one."

Beverly died in 2008. "She had cancer," Thomas told him, pointing to his abdomen. "She's strong, but she had to give up." During that first meeting, he and Beverly's grandson talked for hours. He stood; Thomas rocked back and forth in his wheelchair as they spoke, nervously keeping time. "She always thought about us when she should have been taking care of herself," he told him, echoing a familiar trope of sacrifice and selflessness Beverly would often use, sometimes simply as a way to steer a conversation if it began to move in a direction she did not want or could not tolerate. He told Thomas how he returned to Baltimore to find Beverly, how he had written about his grandmother's struggle with illness and the complicated problems that surrounded her conditions, and how they had stayed in contact long after Thomas and his siblings had been taken from her. Laughing, her grandson told him, "Even after she passed, it was like we all thought she was gonna get better. She always did."

His own thoughts were still very much of her as present and alive—for years after her death, she remained a living, acting figure in his writing, forever passing between the thresholds of health and illness, without the benefit of knowing about her death to close the loop. Since his time reconnecting with Beverly's grandson, as well as her other two grandchildren and her youngest son, he has been reconsidering what it means to return, to recuperate, and in no small way to reassess the years between his last time seeing and talking with Beverly and her passing.

He marches down paths that he thought he had already traveled—he returns to Beverly, following (having followed) and retracing steps through her clinic visits, hospitalizations, and the care of others.

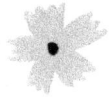

Beverly marched with him.

He was continually surprised by the manner in which Beverly's memory of events would be remade through the different ways those events were described to him, over and over, like a repeating pattern. Beverly would repeat herself often, but each time there was something added, subtracted, or substituted. There was no sameness. He learned from an early point that he was not always welcome to participate in Beverly's remembering. Beverly needed an interlocutor, but one who would quietly follow her story without much intrusion, someone to stand nearby and to listen or see and record. In a real sense her speech was an experiment. Their conversations were a way for her to assert and sometimes insist on meaning in the middle of testing what that meaning could do.

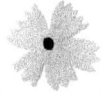

Beverly seemed to reoccupy

        her own story with each telling.

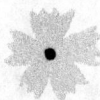

Care.

Care is a conundrum.[2] It is something Beverly gave and received; it is the version of herself told to herself and told to him and others.

Care validates relationships and justifies actions. It is a currency of relatedness, exchanged, cherished, emptied of value, horded, exhausted.

Care is the image of her and the image maker; her failings and his, held up against the horrible realities of the bodily, the social, the racialized, and the derided. To return to the words of Christina Sharpe, care offered "disaster and possibility," asserting a violence faintly recognized, which demanded to be exceeded in order for her to be.[3]

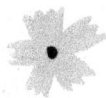

Beverly's eldest son was extremely ill.

Despite years of estrangement, several visits between Beverly and her son in the hospital began to mend the relationship. His first meeting with Beverly's son was when her son came to visit his children, whom Beverly looked after. At the time, he was filled with nervous energy, almost manic. But in the visits that followed, he lost several pounds, appearing gaunt. Beverly described his appearance as "gloom and doom," like he was "already passed."

Once, while they were talking, the phone rang and Beverly answered it. It was this son, who was in the hospital. He asked for money, but she told him just to concentrate on getting better. She was exasperated but told him that she loved him and hung up. "He will call back later," she said. She says that when she was last in the hospital, after she had fallen down her front steps, her bedside phone rang. It was her son with the same request. Dryly, she says that it feels like she's living the same day again and again.

Even though things had improved, Beverly maintained a powerful resentment toward her eldest son and his wife for leaving three grandchildren in her charge through a court-ordered custodianship—one child in a wheelchair, and the younger brother and sister victims of sexual abuse at the hands of their parents' friends, with whom the parents had been abusing drugs. At the same time, Beverly expended great energy to care for her middle son, to help him get to the Moore HIV clinic at the Johns Hopkins Hospital for treatment and to meet with his case manager. Care was offered, and care was withheld. Perhaps the most jarring example of this was when Beverly said at some point that her eldest son and his wife had died. What was striking was the matter-of-fact way this information was conveyed. This, like any number of other topics, was offered and simultaneously closed for further discussion. So he was surprised months later to see her son and daughter-in-law at a family picnic, very much alive.

He had to ask.

She smiled as she told him, "Some people pass before their time."

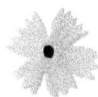

Before your time.

To be placed in passing. In the moment her attitude was somehow unsurprising. She would often rehearse the details of encumbrance the grandchildren presented—children abused and discarded by her son and daughter-in-law. At other times she would insist, "These babies came to me, a blessing." Care was an excuse, an action, and a place where actions would retreat when threatened, or spent.

Beverly acted through the plural character of relationships, even when the tissue of those relationships was stretched dangerously thin.

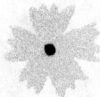

He attempts to record these moments

in the correct tense, in the fullness of that word,

   one that allows the movement of time to

appear as fully as the damage inflicted in the

   moral field of relations in a single instant

(including the damage felt and perpetrated by the

   author without the opportunity for repair).

How terrible, this ethics of the everyday, when it is lived.[4] Tense is not incidental. It is telling that Thomas, Beverly's grandson, said, "She's strong" (in the simple present), rather than using the past tense, "She was strong," even years after her death. Care is the management of tense. Beverly passed and remains present. Her son passes, returns, and will eventually pass again the following year, never to return.

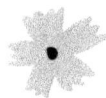

Some people pass before their time.

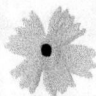

Fixing, to fix.

Maybe Beverly's grandchildren were a burden and a blessing, but to be sure, care moved in both directions, as Thomas from his wheelchair helped Beverly manage her medications and the younger children cooked for the entire family. She says she brought them back from the brink of death. Beverly's grandchildren now perform a different kind of care in their adulthood, as they tell (keep) her story after her death, following her own telling as they discuss his notes and writing with him since his return. She fixed them, and as an action of care, they fix her now—to correct her, fix or hold her in place, the act of fixity. They bring her back from the brink of death.

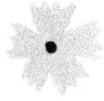

The image of Beverly is found between two moments

in time, between a succession of images she

would create of and for herself, offered to him,

asserted as a way to overwrite something that

came before, to run the present into the past

and smother it, to lose it in the dissolve.

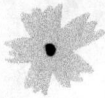

In cinema the dissolve overlaps two shots

to denote the passage of time; it is not

   a double exposure but the absorption

between two equal qualities to facilitate transition.

The dissolve is an effective technical device because it allows us to step (for a moment) out of time, which by now has formed our habits of see-ing time move. Some part of the present is overwritten as it slides into the past; but overwriting is not always erasure and can just as easily con-tain some quality of translucency overlaid on events from the past: the potential to dissolve from one point to another without fully accounting for what lies in between.

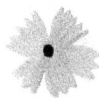

This is where Beverly lived,

        the image of her living, in the tiny,

occulted filaments where her image sparkles.

But unlike the expected duration and form of a film, Beverly risked dissolving altogether—unexpectedly, permanently—never to emerge in the next scene.

    Nothing is guaranteed. Nothing.

A house constitutes a body of images that give mankind proofs or illusions of stability.

GASTON BACHELARD, *The Poetics of Space*

5

A LIVING
ROOM

Sitting in her living room. What occurs here, in this space filled up with her? Once words are spoken, this space recedes to the background; once words are put to bodily experience and the fullness of social relations take shape, this space is overwritten, effaced by the retelling of the things of life that tend to unravel here.

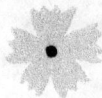

Let me start with an example, a reflection that comes from a short essay titled "Means to Live" by John Berger, on the British photographer Nick Waplington's series Living Room.[1]

Waplington photographed two working-class families, his friends and neighbors in Nottingham, England, for more than a decade, roughly the same length of time I followed Beverly and her family in Baltimore. Berger's reflections on Waplington's photographs are rare because he does not occupy himself with the content of scenes; he does not treat them as tableaux. He is instead drawn to the things that "give expression to the energy of pleasures" in their rendering. His attention rests on what lives "outside the frame" more than the composition within it. Berger writes,

"[Waplington's] photographs are not about captured moments. They are more experiential, constantly evolving over time, commenting on each other, alive. . . . An artist's vision can never be defined just according to what he or she has seen—how he has seen is equally important."[2]

How one has seen and *how scenes comment on each other*—I find these formulations incredibly useful to think with. In the past I followed or attempted to follow individuals as they moved between institutional spaces, between different homes or couches or places where it seemed they were nowhere at all.[3] That attention to motion, to movement in the world, certainly exists in some form in my time with Beverly—chasing her from hospital to hospital, shuttling between family members and friends from neighborhood to neighborhood, tracking her movements through her children and grandchildren as proxies, and even after her death, re-creating these movements in conversations with them, chasing her still. But I was also concerned with dwelling (though *lingering* might be a better, less Heideggerian word) as an element of our encounters. I lingered, caught within a milieu, in this case in the home, and in the living room more specifically. I hung out, which for the ethnographer requires the awareness of intrusion but also requires that feeling to be pushed down, held down, especially in situations when looking away or leaving might be preferable or sensible, when lingering feels wrong. But lingering is necessary; it is the acknowledgment that presence is not the same as a single instance; lingering gives presence—gives sustained contact—its due. By remaining in that living room, I wish to prevent that place from becoming estranged from Beverly's role within it.

Being with her, there, helped to create a record of how her milieu and her psyche were knotted together.

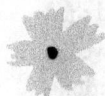

As with many concepts that are put to new use, there's a natural hesitancy about fit.

New uses demand a moment of reflection to consider how the original user may have intended a concept to be used and, more generally, how far concepts can be stretched. Milieu is one. My question of new uses is motivated in part by questions that the physician-philosopher Georges Canguilhem poses in his 1952 essay "The Living and Its Milieu" about the contemporary nature of the category milieu, which for Canguilhem involved a careful accounting of a protracted line of thought through biologists and medical thinkers including Jean-Baptiste Lamarck, Charles

Darwin, Jakob von Uexküll, and Kurt Goldstein.[4] I do not aim to reconstruct that line, only to say that the milieu concept can be easily misappropriated. Perhaps scholars are eager to find new terms for culture (milieu as culture), or to rethink bodily interiority in the guise of experience (a Bernardian line of *milieu intérieur*), or to acknowledge the environment in and through which an organism lives only to more or less dispense with that environment in order to pivot back toward the organism.

On one hand, Canguilhem observed that the notion had become a universal way of capturing both the experience and the existence of living beings, including their composite parts and elements, therefore making it possible to appreciate the idea of milieu as a category of contemporary thought vital to the living understood on different scales. But even a casual reader of Canguilhem's essay will notice one thing straightaway: "the living" resides on one side of the conjunction in the title, the living and *its* milieu. It is not a general milieu concept, not a generic environment, but a milieu proper to *that* organism, to the living—the notion of milieu affirms itself as a central category of contemporary thought, one that is unyielding in its relationship with and about *the living*, including, one could say, "the human."[5]

None of this betrays the genealogy of concepts in biology and philosophy that Canguilhem brings into view, precisely because Canguilhem's view incorporates the problem of individuality, of a cell or something—or someone—else. I find a resource in one thinker essential to Canguilhem's thesis, namely, the neuropsychiatrist Kurt Goldstein, in thoughts outlined in his *The Organism*.[6] Sharing the flavor of Goldstein's conception of milieu, of its pressures on the individual, I take seriously the phantasms and expressions of suffering to which I bore some witness. In this context the mode of anthropological engagement is a form of witnessing, a chosen set of optics that frame and fix a certain exposure of the scene—a scene that enfolds moments of madness as seen in relations to others and to space, to the "ensemble of variables" and the "entourage of living beings" found there.[7] The organism finds itself in a contest of demands and, when sick or threatened, submits to these demands, moves within them, and forms new relationships with and within its milieu. As Canguilhem reads Goldstein, "A life that affirms itself against the milieu is a life already threatened.... A healthy life, confident in its existence, in its values, is a life of flexion, suppleness, almost softness."[8]

A life, soft, plastic, but not gentle. When Beverly could no longer walk up and down the stairs to her bedroom because of pain and shortness of breath, the living room became her bedroom. The life of the home happened there. Her mother slept in a chair, and her preteen grandson often slept in a cramped crib meant for a toddler. The room was constantly configured and reconfigured based on her functioning, on her needs and disappearing autonomy.

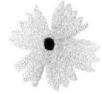

Beverly's living room is a large room

        situated in the front part of her row house.

The front door opens directly into the room. A dining room is to one side; it is unusable as a dining room, filled with boxes and old clothes. Her living room is more than its four walls; so much lives, returning to Berger, "outside the frame." It is cigarette smoke, chemical disinfectants, stale urine, television chatter, and the muffled sounds of neighbors arguing.

Beverly would hole up in the living room on a couch or chair, situated so she could recline and watch things frying or boiling in the kitchen, her eyelids heavy, burners open on the stove. How had she never been engulfed in flames? Her living room appears in the background of my notes, banal as the weather, a medium through which life happens. It was sunny, humid, rainy, or cool. It was morning or early evening. Such and such was there; the conversation went like this or that. I asked questions, scribbled notes, most of them indecipherable, almost as a way of forgetting or forestalling a return to that place until I had some distance or perspective, hazarding a return. We talked about her health, the health of her children and others. On the surface, the structure of these notes over years amounts to little. But these otherwise trivial scenes had the power to saturate deeply, a stain that would reappear, reassert itself unexpectedly, persistent, perhaps even mutually corrosive within the relationship.

A few years after her death, her grandson casually tells me that once, when he was very small, she forced him along with his younger sister and brother into her makeshift bed and began to cover them in blankets and sheets and duvets, and eventually even bath towels. They were tucked in so tightly they could not move. The two younger siblings liked the game at first, and he tells me he, too, felt there was something reassuring about the weight of the heavy blankets. But even as a small child, he knew to wiggle his arms enough to give his younger siblings room to breathe. The younger siblings eventually became scared, and he worried that they would suffocate—something justified when Beverly whispered not to let them (an unnamed them) hear you breathing. It was hot and humid, and Beverly had closed the windows and shades.

And then it stopped.

They were under those blankets for what he described as hours. She eventually ran out of things to pile on top of them. His sister had peed herself, and they wormed out. They found Beverly slumped in a chair, asleep with the television on.

I imagined this scene in the room where I had spent so many hours of nothing. It filled my absence of seeing. My aim is not to link these scenes to some clinical or social concern, at least not directly, but rather to consider the site where distress asserts itself in new terms, in a new relationship to the demands of milieu, a place of immediate demands, still rife with memory. It also needs to be clear that these scenes were always tangled with dozens of other scenes, other pressures, so that if taken cumulatively, they seem routine or almost trivial. They are events that get recorded as nonevents. Even her nonvoluntary short-term psychiatric hospitalizations were always, in the time that I knew her, the by-products of trips to the emergency room for other reasons (problems managing her diabetes, headaches or back pain), events bound up with other events.

And then the milieu would shift, and she within it, a different momentum in the moments of crisis and chaos and longing and confusion—I would leave and return to something wholly different.

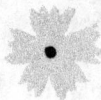

In his essay on the milieu, Canguilhem

evokes the Pascalian interpretation of

   the environment as mi-lieu, *middle:*

the organism is middle, *that is, itself a center.*[9]

The organism does not simply reside there; it draws everything toward itself, wrapping the milieu around itself, as its center. The living room as milieu shrunk around Beverly, even as it made demands on her, pulling in things and spaces beyond that space. Berger saw Waplington's photographs as affirmative and cohesive despite the poverty and social insecurity in which his families lived: the living room offered a means to live. In Beverly's living room I saw an uneasy lack of cohesion and fleeting affirmation—a heady mix of dullness, joy, sorrow, care and its opposite, but still a means to live. And like Waplington's photographs, these ethnographic scenes are not a few captured moments that vacillate between light and dark but rather images of moments that seem to be, to quote Berger again, "commenting on each other, alive." They are the places and substances of living. In the end, I wonder how these lesser milieus might stand up against grander currents of contemporary thought. I wonder where coming apart finds lodging.

what has drowned, has drowned.

She will not return. The headless sky

unseals and aches for us, mother and sister

caught upon the steel hook of its memory

SAFIYA SINCLAIR, "In Childhood,
Certain Skies Refined My Seeing"

6

THOUGHTS OF SUICIDE

Not dark, but sun-drenched. The gathering of a life, of birthdays and mindlessness and fears and passions and failings, tucked away into a few seconds, a single moment.

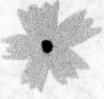

To end, what can be returned to the void?

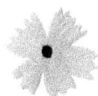

One jerk of the wheel and off the

      bridge that connects Southwest Baltimore

to the edge of Cherry Hill.

It was long; the guardrails were low, at least low enough for a car to jump them with a little speed. The midafternoon traffic was always thin. The sidewalks were broad, but it was rare to see people crossing the bridge on foot. Cherry Hill and Brooklyn were islands ferried mostly by bus or car. Unbuckling the seatbelt, his final gesture before committing, before leaning on the accelerator.[1] *Why wear a seatbelt at all?* So rule-bound.

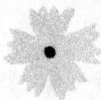

The car would touch the surface

of the water and crumple.

There is nothing constant about water. Its surface—viscous, alchemical, soft or stone—waits to receive. Playing on a riverbank as a kid, accidently slipping under moving sheets of ice, a friend pulling his limp body out of the water by the hood of his sweatshirt, soaked and leadened, the water a thick brown jelly and slush. Contact opens a register of the water's materiality previously unknown, a rush of new knowledge and then the enveloping cold or heat, the shock of yellow and white, tunnel vision and ringing, and the hope of disappearance, digestion.

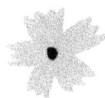

Would the sensation of

falling be familiar?

The joy of a stomach turning somersaults as a child, after mustering the courage to leap from high into the black water below, the sharp sting of water forcing its way up his nose, a victory. *The earned sting of letting go.* Cauterizing, the singe of ammonia in the nostrils carried on the breeze from the fertilizer factory behind his childhood home. Bans of piss-warm water mixing with cooler, deeper water, green yellow brown, small sunfish darting, silver in the sunlight that penetrates a primordial soup of algae and protozoa and beginnings. Beneath the surface, his eyes open, a flirtation with panic at the edge of disorientation. Sprays of memory, of summer's sun pushing through leaves, the sounds of laughing screams and splashes and the smell of musty towels and the pleasure of soggy shoes.

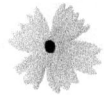

Filthy. Joyous.

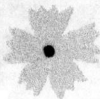

Was nostalgia possible in the

instant before the end, or

maybe it was the only thing?

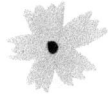

On the side of the road is a collection

of trash amassed by car tires and wind

and poor drainage, trash and bottles, gravel,

small holdouts of dirty snow and slurry.

Harbor water the color of Yoo-hoo swells with the tide and hints at the water's depth.

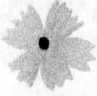

Trips to the back stoop of his row

house to smoke interrupt internet

searches for ways to end.

He is stretched thin, so thin. To-do lists and night sweats. Dreaming of carcinomas. Thoughts churn, but not productive thoughts, just the look of thought that amounts to nothing, an aesthetic of productivity culti-vated over time and by example, performed in correct gestures, the right words chosen and said on cue.

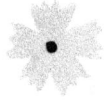

Driving, the glare of the ugly winter sun

                    revealing water spots and greasy smudges

on the inside of the windshield.

Was there enough Windex in the world for a windshield like this? He is carried on a wave of guilt for caring so much about things so small.

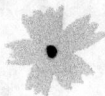

Pain. There's a scene in Stanley Kubrick's

Paths of Glory *(1957) where three French soldiers*

in their trench bunker the night before battle

chat about how they would prefer to die.

Their rationale (for a bullet, for shrapnel, for an injury to the head or the chest) hinges on the sensation of pain and the awareness of death. Was it better to know pain while awaiting death? To linger a little longer, alert, knowing your demise? Or was it better to disappear in an instant, without pain and the knowledge of death it brings? In the end the three are shot for cowardice. There's a lesson here.

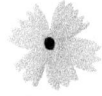

Deliberation.

A self-inflicted gunshot wound requires a gun, something politically horrible for him. *Knife*: the thought nauseates him. *Pills*: vomit. *Opiates*: too
much time to think before unthinking, too much awareness. *Asphyxia-
tion*: the fear is survival, brain damage, a life with cognitive impairment—
spending weeks worrying about the cost of survival. *How petty? So, so
vain.*

But pettiness and vanity together act as a kind of life support.

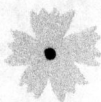

Years later he is still woozy thinking about all

that was hidden from friends and family,

the self-indulgence and his nearness to the end.

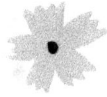

A car accident.

No note. The loss of control. *Is it not the truth, losing control?* Accidents insulate against the satisfaction of others, not knowing the will to death or simply dying?

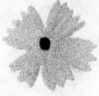

Pitiful.

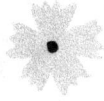

Every trip to Beverly's house

possessed flashes of the same.

Small rehearsals. It was a dreaded drive. These thoughts rarely accompanied him on his trip home; they were reserved for the moments before whatever waited to be endured. The drive from Beverly's home to his home, from a house on fire to one filled with artificial warmth.

Find a distraction.

Go for a run.

Maybe stop eating for a while, to enjoy the prize of hunger.

Voice hoarse from too much smoke and stomach acid.

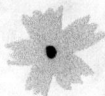

There is something about the mélange

of anger, sentimentalism, and loathing

that keeps a person perched on the edge,

the pharmakon of anthropology.

Writing went nowhere. The twilight of a relationship. Bracing for the embarrassment of failure after years of study, of smarts, turned inside out, his desire to crush and to be crushed. Returning again and again to a house, to a woman who turned her own screw, whose health problems were some kind of refuge for him it seemed.

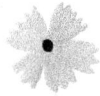

In art school a friend committed suicide

                        immediately after the death of Kurt Cobain.

He was drunk. He set up a circle of CDs and fan paraphernalia and shot himself in the head, a violently ironic homage. Could he really have been making a joke? In the months leading up to his death he had become more and more self-destructive, mostly sex, but also drugs and small acts of nonsense like hurdling the third rail of the "L" tracks at night, demanding others do the same, bound together in this stupid, spontaneous rite of passage. He channeled Robert Rauschenberg in his wild art. *Goat.* "To fuck like a goat," he would say. He was desperate to connect to something, anything, primitive and profane. He found out he was HIV positive. He was lonely and angry and funny and on fire.

He was from Texas. His friends used Tupperware to collect pieces of buckshot and brain tissue they had picked out of the wall of his home and brought them back to Chicago for his wake. In the aftermath they drank and mourned, stomach cramps not from the alcohol but from the anxiety of not knowing where to place the loss of this friend. It was impossible to unclench. On the way home he and others stopped by a diner. The mood worsened, and he was attacked for not being sufficiently shit-faced and grief-stricken. They harassed a waitress, threw loose change, and he left wheezing and coughing and crying as he walked up Belmont Avenue in the rain.

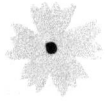

Beverly's house was a refuge.

He could sit and smoke with her. It didn't matter. It was a place falsely shielded from external scrutiny. She knew scrutiny. But it was a place to give in to the everything of her.

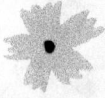

Fieldwork was a forest into which he could wander and disappear.

How many paces into the wilderness before the romance of desolation dissolved?

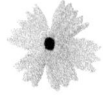

His, a sudden, piercing self-violence.

Hers, a low snarl of violences outside of her, folded into her.

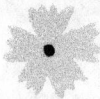

His nightmare of a coma after

a botched attempt to end: Could there

be a more perfect picture of hell?

Catheter, eyes taped shut, mouth stupidly open, confused loved ones in a state of irritated pity. *Serves him right.* His thoughts stir him into consciousness.

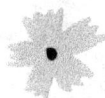

He writes this now, something he could never

      say then, even in a dream, to exorcise these

thoughts that were passengers during fieldwork,

      before cutting the wheel and tasting brine,

a split second of revulsion and relief.

I embark on a voyage of seeing.

HIROSHI SUGIMOTO, *Seascapes*

[. . .]

7

I am a great admirer of the photographer Hiroshi Sugimoto, especially the series he began in 1980 titled *Seascapes*. Each photograph in *Seascapes* is split along a horizon separating sea and sky, two complementary atmospheres of water and air in tones of black and white and silver and gray. The composition is always the same, but the quality of the sky and water is infinitely varied. Take *North Pacific Ocean, Ohkurosaki, neg. 581* (2013), its water lit from some engine sunken in the depths, its surface illuminated glass reflecting a sky of terraced clouds. Or *Bay of Sagami,*

Kaikoh, neg. 579 (2011), completely blurry, shrouded under a blanket, a flashlight against the surface of flesh; or *Bay of Sagami, Atami, neg. 503* (1997), which inverts sky and sea, pitch-black night pushing down on an ocean of diluted phosphorescence; or *Lake Superior, Cascade River, neg. 570* (1995), its flat sky and flat sea, both so matched in whiteness that the division is nearly impossible to distinguish, small black wrinkles of waves the only things that break the smoothness of the water, without their disruption the image possessing only faint depth; or *Bass Strait, Table Cap, neg. 465* (1997), its undifferentiated white sky resting against the ink-black water of hidden Leviathans. Despite always dividing the plane of the image evenly, the horizons in some photographs appear quite close, and in others they stretch out for a terrible distance—what would it take to reach this threshold between sky and water, to meet that divide with touch?

I give examples, but each photograph is unique; there is no one quality that binds the photographs of *Seascapes*, nothing that forms a standard image from which the others deviate. I never imagined these works as an inventory of snapshots taken from Sugimoto's travels; instead I see them as a series of singular photographs that, on one hand, aim to forget the image that came before and, on the other, aim to better capture the same scene or its essence with each successive try.

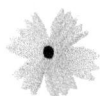

I love these photographs. It is hard to

      ignore their meditative quality,

and for me it is easy to give in to them.

I want to believe these photos were taken not from the shoreline but by the photographer lost at sea; the sea and sky before him having a giant, unseen twin in the sea and sky that surrounds him, unrecorded, out of view but whose weight is felt. Would the image look the same if he spun around quickly in his lifeboat to capture the scene to his back? I like to think there is a mirror to each one of these photographs, infinite degrees of supposed sameness in any single image that would tell a different story of behindness, adjacentness, in that moment of capture of what lies ahead.

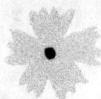

One photograph in particular,

Ligurian Sea, Saviore, neg. 390 *(1993)*,

has repeatedly taken me in.

The atmosphere is hazy, a dull fog pulling all of the gray tones to a common center: the sea and sky want to dissolve into one gray. Waves on the water are reminders that nothing is static, nothing is staged, but more than this, nothing of what this image captures will remain. *Churning.* But the thing that keeps me coming back to this photograph is its horizon, a halo that flips light and dark, pushing the horizon back toward the viewer, back into the water that connects the viewer with that horizon, which simultaneously lifts the horizon into the sky. In the photograph, the horizon is energy that refuses both sky and sea.

I have considered this photograph dozens of times, searching for its trick of inversion. In the strictest sense, this trick, which is not a trick at all, makes this photograph poignant to me; it bruises my sensibilities by revealing to me how much I rely on the clear horizon of other photographs for comfort, my eye returning to their horizons to rest, relying on the divide and distance to explain to me my point of view.[1]

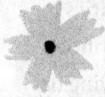

I wish I could put words to the quality

of difference in Beverly's story of herself

and my story of her.

I wish I could say plainly what distinguishes one horizon from the next, because maybe that would explain why certain images assert themselves more than others. By now I have accepted that the protagonist of this story is between us. Maybe what I am looking for is the quality of connection between certain images, between moments of uneven intensity. I believe some images are worth returning to over others, reasons for which I cannot often explain, but they share the same line in the middle of the image that divides the sea and sky. When is it ever not the case that we feel our way through difference; when do we not make choices that are hard to account for, to which we find it impossible to apply a rationale to explain our tastes or desires?

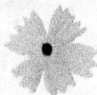

The horizons in Sugimoto's photographs

hover between life and death, standing in for

something that has yet to be filled, an ellipsis.

I feel drawn to this place, a place of in betweens. I wonder if the thing that is poignant about the image, piercing about an image—my version of Roland Barthes's *punctum*—can be found not in one image but between images, not despite the image but because they are always more than one. Even when one moment asserts itself, dominates my point of view, perhaps dwelling with the substance that hangs between this moment and other moments offers awareness that "the unknown can affirm life with negative shapes."[2] Is the sea-in-between a substance that allows us to drift or invites us to drown?

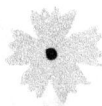

For so long I mistook impermanence

and singularity for repetition.

Her words and gestures are a constant drift, in my record of them, in the images I have amassed. I do not have a different point of view on the same sea, but new seas with a common horizon.

How then does light return to the world after the eclipse of the sun? Miraculously. Frailly. In thin stripes. It hangs like a glass cage. It is a hoop to be fractured by a tiny jar. There is a spark there. Next moment a flush of dun. Then a vapour as if earth were breathing in and out, once, twice, for the first time.

VIRGINIA WOOLF, *The Waves*

8

BREATHING FEELS LIKE A FALSEHOOD

To be with Beverly, a rhythm starts to make itself known, rising and falling: the meter is like breathing, moments that are short of breath—wheezing, coughing from a long struggle with emphysema, and the breathlessness brought on by chronic obstructive pulmonary disease—and other moments, lungs filled, tissue stretched, holding for an instant before pushing out air and endless speech.

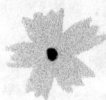

The mood darkens.

He watches as an intense panic comes over Beverly as she struggles to catch her breath, heaving, desperate to move through this struggle, a terrific dread, the thought that getting through this may not happen, a terror that passed between them, a panic met by his own horror at witnessing her distress. Even now when he recalls this moment he feels his own dyspnea, a shortness of breath that requires deliberate movements, forcing a change in tempo, slowing down the frames that at greater speed blur to smooth over this moment. He slows in order to clock each frame. There is no easy way out of this.

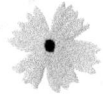

The image of Beverly is dictated by respiration,

dictated by the individual rhythms of life

that shape our ideas of what life is and

how we are able to conceptualize it.[1]

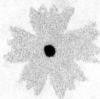

There is so much doubt about the breath,

even when no virus is present to

        inflame the lungs, no one to press his knee

against her windpipe.

Breathing in the political moment of this writing is a locus of distrust, something to question and to be extinguished, at the heart of a politics of erasure.

    It is impossible to think breathing without thinking the conditions of vital difference, to think with the conditions of the world that are taken in unevenly on breath, and returned.[2]

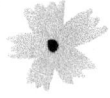

He holds her hand while her mother

calls an ambulance.

No one else is home.

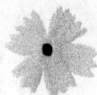

He is emptied out except for the thought

that this is it, her end; he is witness

to a scene she predicted so many times.

Her hand is so dry. He holds it tighter, attempting to match her grip. His hand is a messenger. His body as an instrument, so paltry, but still he presses against the surface of his subject, pushing into her, hoping something is transmitted.

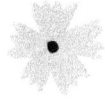

Holding her hand.

When she inhales, her eyes widen.

He can hear her chest crackle. He imagines a plastic valve pinched with each gasp. He rubs his thumb over the hand he is holding. He uses his futile telepathy to communicate a thought he does not believe. This will pass. This will be OK.

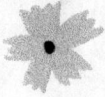

Pneuma *and* psyche.

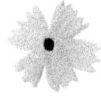

He thinks of living organisms in the absence

of oxygen—of fermentation, of

*Louis Pasteur's life without air (*la vie sans l'air*).*

Beverly is fermenting, agitated and changed. No, she is suffocating.

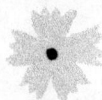

Where is she in all of this?

He does not see her in her eyes.

Her mother is on the phone, angrily asking the dispatcher when the ambulance will arrive.

This is not the first time the ambulance has come for Beverly in the time he has known her. Why will she speak of this moment with such cold indifference weeks from now?

She forecasted her passing, but this time, like all the rest he has known, she will pull back from the brink and regain her breath.

She will return, but a reprieve from nothing.

How can she regard these moments, their breathlessness, as monotonous? How could he? Was she not feeling the special force of this moment in the moment? Was it not different from the rest, more urgent than the last? Was it monotony that she scorned or fate?

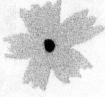

Lollygagging.

Where is the ambulance? The minutes barricade themselves against us.

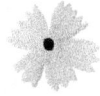

Thomas Mann's The Magic Mountain

　　　　　　details the phantasms of tuberculosis,

the sanatorium, and the kinships formed around

　　　　　　and within a sickness of the lungs,

where ultimately the disease-subject is borne out.

This is evident as Mann's Hans Castorp struggles to apply meaning to the body under the conditions of sickness as a particular form of life:

> This body, then, which hovered before his, this individual and living I, was a monstrous multiplicity of breathing and self-nourishing individuals, which, through organic conformation and adaptation to special ends, had parted to such an extent with their

essential individuality, their freedom and living immediacy, had so much become anatomic elements.

    …

Thus far pathology, the theory of disease, the accentuation of the physical through pain; yet, in so far as it was the accentuation of the physical, at the same time accentuation through desire. Disease was a perverse, a dissolute form of life. And life? Life itself? Was it perhaps only an infection, a sickening of matter? Was that which one might call the original procreation of matter only a disease, a growth produced by morbid stimulation of the immaterial? The first step toward evil, toward desire and death, was taken precisely then, when there took place that first increase in the density of the spiritual, that pathologically luxuriant morbid growth, produced by the irritant of some unknown infiltration; this, in part pleasurable, in part a motion of self-defense, was the primeval stage of matter, the transition from the insubstantial to the substance. This was the fall … the next step on the reckless path of the spirit dishonored.[3]

Where does this reckless path lead? In this passage, life and disease and drives and death are presented as competing though primordially complementary elements. Here, disease is rendered not as an epistemological problem but as an ontological solution; its "infiltration" is indiscernible from the being of the so-called disease-subject, emerging as a monstrously multiple "I." Similarly, Michel Foucault suggests that the idea of a disease attacking a life must be replaced by the much denser notion of pathological life.[4] Disease, in the world of Mann, can both pervert and preserve life.

It helps a little.

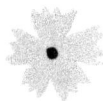

To pervert and preserve life.

The attention to sickness, to the symptom (Beverly's attention and his), enfolds the terms of life, how a life is lived and for whom, complete with the anxiety that is not always made explicit, that she has taken the path of the dishonored or, as Virginia Woolf writes, "become a deserter in the army of the upright."[5]

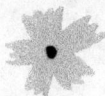

Up the front steps with oxygen,

the paramedics are giants,

or maybe our need shrinks us.

Their swagger is reassuring. They lift Beverly out of the house and off of him. She has gone limp. He releases her and seals himself off from her. He has no urge to follow.

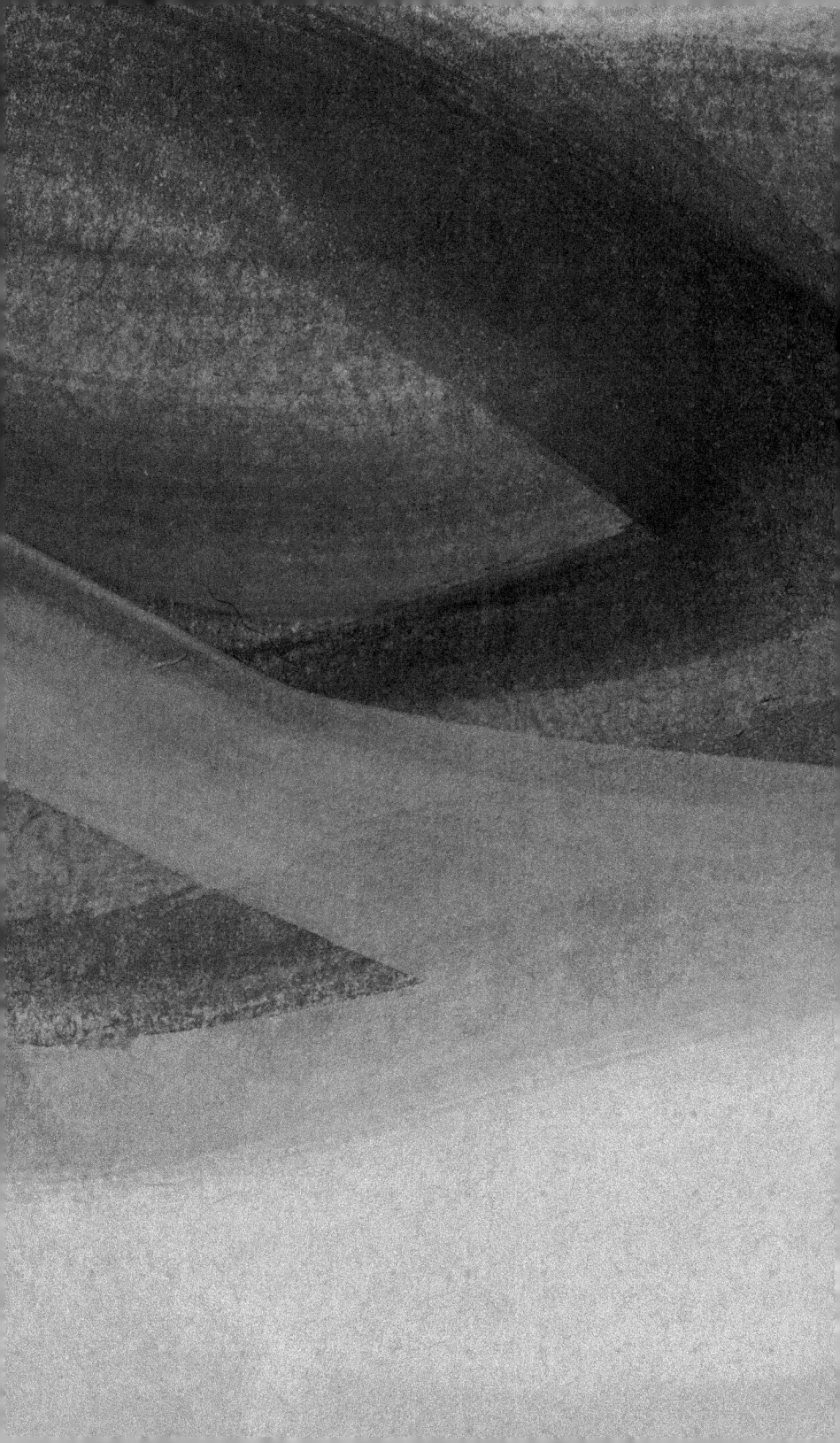

I would be the unhappiest person imaginable, confronted daily with disastrous works crying out with errors, imprecision, carelessness, amateurishness. I *avoided* this punishment *by destroying them*, I thought, and suddenly I took great pleasure in the word *destroying*.

THOMAS BERNHARD, *The Loser*

9

NOTES
ON A
NEW
MORALISM

I have always loved errors. When I was an undergraduate studying painting at the School of the Art Institute of Chicago, one pleasure was to
visit the Prints and Drawings room of the museum. We got to touch
works on paper made by names we admired. We held them in our hands,
amplifying their inviolability and demystifying them all at once. I always
wanted to see work that had been seemingly discarded by the artist,
started but unfinished, works without titles, images obsessed over, line
after line committed until the right grain was found, or not.

I was drawn to the proof of trial and error, the product of inexactitude; I was taken in by the sloppy power of these drawings, their ability to emancipate the artist from any obligation to harmony; I recognized the intrepid and affirmative good found in things not yet fully realized that still somehow remained things.

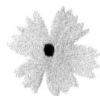

These drawings were, after all, failures.

Despite the astonishing and varied skill demonstrated in their lines, they were not masterworks; they failed to seal themselves off from being any other way—what is a masterwork other than an image that does not allow its viewer's imagination to consider it in another form? It is as it is. My drawings were plastic, eager to be refashioned, even by the viewer in looking.

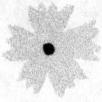

Malleability and the hunger to be corrected:
this is precisely the power of error—error not
*　　　　　as negligence, not as harm produced by*
a series of misguided actions, but instead
*　　　　　a moment captured in a line passed over and*
over again, a lesson of its limit; failure taught
*　　　　　through the satisfying prick of disharmony.*

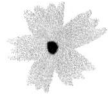

I sensed failure was my object

       long before I found the nerve to name it.

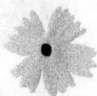

I seek guidance from masters of failure.

There is a lesson in Thomas Bernhard's *Woodcutters*; a narrator, adopting the stance of the casual observer at a terrible, pretentious dinner party, nevertheless inserts himself into the fray in every cutting comment, slicing himself into the bourgeois social order he is so desperate to stand outside of, tethered to the tiny world he seeks to dismantle; or, perhaps especially, a lesson of failure is found in Bernhard's memoir, *Gathering Evidence and My Prizes*, wherein he pulls himself apart in passage after passage, a call and response of confession and self-criticism. For Bernhard, there is no mystery to his own deconstruction; it is an origin story.[1]

Osamu Dazai's awareness of his unmaking is made even more explicit than Bernhard's in Dazai's novel *No Longer Human*. Like a detective, or an ethnographer, his narrator pieces together the past of a man through three photos and three notebooks that he finds, a man who as a child was precocious, self-involved, a bad student who was not corrupted but was a corruptor. *No Longer Human* is unsentimental; it is the story of a child who becomes a man who finds no redemption for himself, a book filled with little flickers of regret, and, for Dazai, a book that is wholly autobiographical (the subtitle of the book is "Confessions of a Faulty Man").

Osamu Dazai's characters are like instruments that are unable to perform the task they were designed for, even as they describe perfectly the task, masters of awareness of expectations external to themselves. They view at a distance the world of which they were meant to be a part; unlike Bernhard's characters, Dazai's tainted protagonist uses this distance to see with crystal clarity the great expanse of human relations and acceptable actions, a world to which his characters are tied through lines of moral failure.[2]

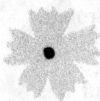

There is something fundamental for Beverly's

story at the intersection of awareness and upheaval,

something Georges Canguilhem describes in

health's genealogy in the history of thought.[3]

In his essay "Health: Popular Concept and Philosophical Questions," Canguilhem traces a genealogy of concepts from Hippocrates to Immanuel Kant to Kurt Goldstein on the quiet potency of bodily silence as vital instruction between health and illness, taking a line from his most famous teacher, the surgeon René Leriche: "Health is life lived in the silence of the organs." But then, maybe even uncharacteristically, Canguilhem turns to Henri Michaux's Nietzschean appraisal of this disquiet:

Just as the body (its organs and its functions) has been mainly known and revealed not by the prowess of the strong, but by the disorders of the sick, the weak, the infirm, and the wounded (health being silent, the source of an immensely erroneous impression that everything goes along by itself), it is the disturbances of the spirit, its dysfunctions, that will be my teachers.[4]

Michaux reverses the value of health altogether, asking if its silence teaches us anything at all about life.[5] I hear Bernhard and Dazai in Canguilhem's quote by Michaux, their refusal to allow failure to open a path to some moral overcoming, eschewing a version of humanity that uses the darkness of collapse to understand by contrast the superficial light of good. After all, in the story of a life, what lesson are we looking for?

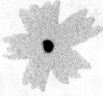

I tried to read to her.

Is it right? Is it okay?

She tells me I can say anything. She has no patience for words repeated back to her. Recitation is poison to her. But I try.

I have always fought the temptation to provide a sense of continuity in my treatment of Beverly's words and actions, a sense of continuity that may have been absent when I first encountered those words and actions. I have avoided coherence in retelling where there is little or no coherence to be found. Beverly would tell me about family members, people outside of her home who depended upon her financially and emotionally, people she felt close to, and then sometime later, suddenly, these family members would disappear from her stories, or I would learn from her son or mother that they died or had lost touch with the family years ago, or were unknown. I held on to my sense of loss and confusion, and I held these contradictions up to Beverly like a greasy mirror. It is little wonder she had no interest in looking.

What to do with tarnished moments? I want to push back against the idea that Beverly is found only in the dim flicker of certain events, to believe, as Karl Ove Knausgaard writes, that she "was not concentrated in individual events but spread over such large areas that it was not possible to comprehend them in anything other than abstract terms."[6] But still, what to do with these events that leave individual marks? Where do I place the moment that we sat there uncomfortably in her living room while she struggled to remember my name after years of knowing me? She smiled, on the verge of tears, completely lost.

She would talk at length about truth, about wanting to be true. This was one reason I insisted on reading my words to her. Truth, however, had nothing to do with the accuracy of my notes or writing. It was something baser. It was something that in moments of paranoia she felt needed testing.

Once, she wanted me to eat something she had cooked. I had eaten many things that she had cooked, but in this case she was oddly unrelenting from the moment I came in the door. I did in fact relent and was ill for days after. I thought it might just have been simple food poisoning, but it became clear that it was something more, as she later spoke of the usefulness of truth serum to find out the answers to questions others refused to answer. I asked whether she had ever given someone truth serum, and she grinned and shook her head no.

I still hoped for some truth to pass between us.

Her stories are filled with ghosts, people from the past who advise and torment her, cruel white men who are quietly murdered without recourse. Police who come into her room at night only to watch her sleep, or who stand outside her window. She hurls insults at passing cars from her porch as we sit talking, her profanity and bubbly affect doing constant battle.[7]

I serpentined in and out of Beverly, in and out of these moments with her, something that taken altogether might be called context. But she emancipated me from the trap of harmony long ago.

Together we dragged things down.

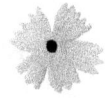

So we descend.

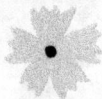

There are pictures of the world that are

worth disrupting, indices of how to live found

        in places of privilege and controlled access

so natural to judgment that they inform

        the vital as much as the social.[8]

I hate the idea of creating an image of Beverly that would fail to acknowledge a system that already judges her in vital-social terms, that judges her on the basis of living, on the fact that she dares to possess life at all, a flattened picture of a poor Black woman in America. I worry about how natural this picture is already.

    I also worry about stopping. The privilege not to finish what is started: the failure to risk anything after she risked so much.

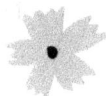

Beverly cared.

She also held resentments and withheld care. Others might do the same in situations of poverty and need, but this is about her. She was cruel. She loved. Poverty forced Beverly's hand. She made decisions about which of her prescriptions to fill based on limited resources. She shared medications with her mother to save money. Unpaid bills and spotty adherence to treatment frayed relationships between Beverly and those upon whom she depended in various medical environments.

She passed bad checks in more ways than one.

Care is a resource, but one that was continually depleted. Beverly tells me, "I can get sick, but then I need to take care of others, and everybody get they turn." But sometimes there is nothing to return.

Nothing is guaranteed. Nothing.

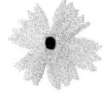

What kinds of contortions are necessary to step out

of tropes of suffering in anthropological writing,

to see what might be found in a different light?

But to do so is to bend, to turn oneself crooked. Still it surprises me that the posture toward suffering in anthropology has resulted in so many straight backs. I am twisted.

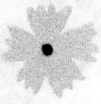

What is a relationship without

the shame attached to it?

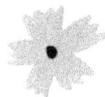

A world filled with so many failings

might lead us to consider whether or not

we have been duped by morality altogether,

or perhaps, more precisely, by its normativity.

Maybe a good place to start is to acknowledge that there is nothing about our humanity—about the character of relations—that is guaranteed.[9] This is critical, not because it acknowledges the hollowing out of a subject by the world but because it alerts us to what might be poured, instead, into that space.[10] I see sin in the appeal of virtue to domesticate suffering and loss. And in the case of Black families in the United States, does the appeal of resilience not offer subtle hints of what these families ought and ought not do—the paternalisms of so-called moral laboratories?[11] Even in the history of the Black body, where humanness is founded in terms of recuperation from other forms, there is nothing given.[12] The world is a hollowing place, surely, but how utterly corrosive is the refusal to absorb the negative?

Nothing is guaranteed. Nothing.

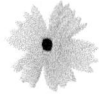

I step onto the porch of her house years after

      she passed, trying to explain to the new tenants

what I have trouble committing to paper.

I am there because I desire contact. I steal looks over their shoulders into what was once Beverly's home.

I tried to engage in the labor of knowing her, but Beverly engaged so often in a kind of counterlabor, defensive and reinventive, obscuring and hopeful. Still, this essay masks the defects of that labor even while attempting to acknowledge them. Maybe some of this has to do with the available ways of representing. Maybe some of this has to do with exhaustion. There is always too much to say without much acknowledgment of the limits of what should be said, or not said, with no way to log that restraint.[13]

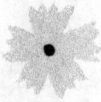

"Illness is the great confessional."[14]

I do not think Virginia Woolf wrote these words with the Christian act of truth telling—confession as a source and technology of truth—in mind. Her account leaves very little room for absolution.[15] Illness may be the great confessional, but not because it invites truth. Whatever comes pouring out is the product of exhaustion, "childish outspokenness," an exorcism of all that has been colonized and taken up residence in the subject.[16] All that was hoped for dissolved long ago. What remains, what can be said, has abandoned its relation to expectation, has formed a relationship with the negative because that is what remains. Anne Boyer writes:

> Living takes the shape of the effort to exist. In the long night of the *effort to exist's* case file, each hour recedes into a lack of energy to achieve a measure of that hour's length. Everything is tired—that's how it gets exhausted—and a person trying to take notes on this writes, "I'm exhausted," because they are too tired to put down their pen.[17]

Poetry can repair no loss, but it defies the space that separates. And it does this by its continual labour of reassembling what has been scattered.

JOHN BERGER, "The Hour of Poetry"

10

BLACK
FIGURINE

I spent a summer's day searching for an object that meant something to me, or came to mean something to me after the fact. I spent a day reassembling what had been scattered.

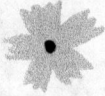

I start in the basement.

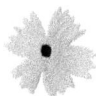

I suppose I want to recover the figurine because

        it is a substitute for Beverly, a kind of avatar,

something to hold for the lack of her.

My search is an exercise to recover something about Beverly that she never possessed—not the object itself, it was real, sitting there, gathering dust; my effort is to recover its character: diminutive, passive, sentimental, available, predictable and constant. The figurine is a channel to Beverly in death, a double of all the things that she was not.

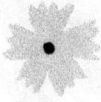

A Black woman with a basket under her arms,

crouched, collecting something from the ground,

in a field, white dress, kerchief—this woman

sat in Beverly's living room.

There are so many ways I tried to code this object—kitsch, antebellum, naive. I searched for the figurine after Beverly's death. Whatever it held, I know its disappearance robs me of something.

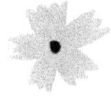

There were other objects in her living room—

reproductions of African masks, plastic flowers

covered in grime in tall painted vases, funeral

notices printed on colored paper with

pictures of family members and friends and

their children (mostly young men, some I

recognize but most I do not), church programs,

so many ashtrays, family portraits.

And then there was the figurine. I notice a small chip exposing the ceramic under its finish; where the enamel is removed, it returns to powder.

Is it a fetish? Michael Taussig writes about the wooden figurines used by Cuna Indian healers from the coasts of Panama and Colombia, powerful objects resembling colonial masters, depictions that overtake their source, together melting the possessor, the object, and the kernel of whatever force hides within.[1] Beverly's figurine was not a simulacrum but a fun-house mirror; its power was its capacity to distort, and it did not give violence but seemed to receive it. The figurine was a votive, a reliquary hiding shards of *sarira*, the distillation of her after her death, awaiting veneration, devotion. Can an object meet the measure of a fetish if it does not play at the edge of falsehood?[2] Beverly's figurine was soft, tamable. Or was this its trick? The term *fetish* moves too near a conclusion, too obvious in its effort to contain and control the object in a word, itself caught in a hierarchy of value.[3]

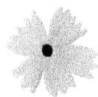

One afternoon I searched for the figurine in

the basement of Beverly's grandson's row house,

a few doors down from where Beverly once lived.

After Beverly's death, her family put her belongings into thirty or so boxes that eventually found their way to Thomas's musty basement. I rummage through each one; her grandson sits behind me, smoking and occasionally offering words of encouragement.

The summer heat has not reached the basement, but the humidity has. I swim in sweat.

I am digging a ditch. Box after box contains the strata of her past that I etch away, really physically *to cut at*.

I am a misguided archeologist, a treasure hunter, desecrating one small tomb at a time.

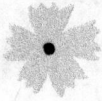

Fat.

I wish I were in better shape. I carry Thomas down the stairs, and then I go back up again to collect his wheelchair. When he needs to use the toilet, we go up the stairs and back down again.

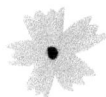

Sinew. *I sort through damp clothes and*

old birthday cards, costume jewelry and

countless tchotchkes, but no figurine.

The clothes are heavy; every fold reveals an odor, the faint smell of urine, mothballs, the body of the last wearer. They are husks, molted skins. I refold and repack the clothes in the boxes as best I can. There is nothing neutral about touching her clothes. It is hard not to feel near to her and contaminated by her even in her absence, the unwanted magic of contact.

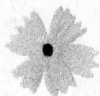

The figurine has a history.

It was her mother's mother's, purchased at a flea market in North Caro-lina a few years before the family moved north. I know this because I asked once. But this history offers no clues to the quality of this object, nothing about the closeness with which it was held or admired, or what other objects may have been held close or closer. But it reminds me of something; it pushes into Beverly, an imprint of her. It is something I can press into her.

The figurine is a hollowed-out space, an empty mold that turns John Berger's words inside out: "The task was to dismantle the block—to take it apart and lift it off piece by piece," but this dismantling reveals not a weighted form, a fleshy body, bronze or plaster, but only the empty space where a body once was.[4] The things that surround her are the only things that define her, that give her shape.

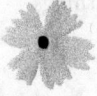

I am in the basement, miserable, still

marveling at the invitation, to be granted access.

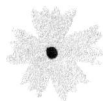

Thievery.

I take moments from the past and abscond with them. I offer nothing in exchange. I say I am searching out opportunities to mend, to suture a wound, but I do so in the absence of a patient, with no say from her (where all speech has been given, where everything that will ever be spoken between us has been spoken), to come to terms with her dying, not as some kind of fantasy of resuscitation but to say something final, finally, at the end of the history of a relationship.

Writing can aspire to reanimate the dead, or an image of the dead, no matter how wearily. But this action leaves little instruction about how to set those images aside once our necromancy is finished—or, as Joan Didion suggests, to let the dead return to photographs on a table.[5] Even after death, a subject moves, she refuses to hold still long enough for the contours of her image to sharpen, apparitions that stay apparitions.[6] The final word is both an end and a declaration of method; it is the theory of how a world is, how a particular cosmology that surrounds a person is legible by making it legible.[7] My ambition is to turn the apparatus of writing into something other than an instrument for telling what we already know, to unbracket the subject and offer the final word as an action of nonmastery, to attend to its (her) ferocity, to reveal by loosening the grip, to become cozy with loss, and perhaps to invite a relationship with the negative.

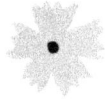

What must it have meant to start writing

about the death of his mother the day

after her passing in October 1977, as

Roland Barthes prepared his course on the topic

of "the Neutral" at the Collège de France?

In one of the early entries in his *Mourning Diary*, Barthes writes, "As soon as someone dies, frenzied construction of the future (shifting furniture, etc.): futuromania." And the following day, "Who knows? Maybe something valuable in these notes?"[8] From the beginning of her end Barthes admits his frenzy to establish meaning and acknowledges the possibility that all this activity might possess little value. The diary, recorded daily on small slips of paper, gave shape to his experience of loss, or rather took shape without closing him off from his grief. It is hard to find a direct influence that his mourning diary may have had on his course—what Roland Barthes called his exercise in "phantasmic teaching"—but there are traces from the diary in his lectures, not in tone but in the way he describes the Neutral as seeking to "outplay the paradigm," to maneuver away from forms of givenness.[9] Was his diary intended to outplay grief or simply to get some purchase on it?[10] The diary was not intended to cup a grief already known. With it he intended to experiment with understanding, to avoid falling into the trap of loss that seems to be waiting for us, something ready-made, something external to us, programmed and ordinary and completely foreign. I believe Barthes's diary sought not to outsmart death but to outsmart the mastery of death, to unthread it, one entry at a time. What his diary amounts to is not the final word on a loss but a word that is his own.[11]

Perhaps the more fundamental problem with the final word has something to do with the anticipation of its form—not through interpretation but through its surplus, the trace of meaning once all is said and done, a gesture of the thing, something in which we participate but which we only really give a little push to help it into the world, and then it is all on its own. Barthes considered the potency of the gesture through his admiration for the paintings of Cy Twombly. He writes, "Let us distinguish the *message*, which seeks to produce information, and the *sign*, which seeks to produce an intellection, from the *gesture*, which produces all the rest (the 'surplus') without necessarily seeking to produce anything."[12]

Twombly *gestures* through lines that are lush, animated; patterns loop and become wild, their forms held on canvas in a way that suggests they could not be anything else, and we experience them in reverse, from their completion traced back through their action.[13] Perhaps to commit to the final word is to commit to a gesture, with the "clumsiness" (*gaucherie*) that Barthes appreciates in Twombly's lines—lines that for Barthes divide life and death.[14] The final word, a gesture, imperfect, made without necessarily seeking to produce anything, produces all the rest.

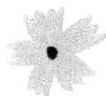

I ask and Thomas tells me that

his aunt knew who took his cousin.

Not taken, "gone off with." He remembers the night I came. His cousin eventually moved to DC after becoming pregnant months later. He tells me his sister lost a baby not long after. In my mind she is still a petite, sleepy-eyed eight-year-old girl.

    I try to explain my feelings from that night. I can't. Why bring this up? Rotten fruit still hanging on a branch of memory waits to be shaken loose, exploding on the ground below, a fetid mess. In whatever form, my private failure still resides in his thoughts (or did I return these thoughts to him?).

So much occurred a few doors down from where we are having this conversation.

I ask, "Why stay?"

"I don't know other places," he tells me.

I suppose I could give the same answer to the question.

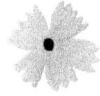

I told Thomas I had a dream

about his grandmother.

In my dream Beverly was hostile toward my writing. "How can you write such things? Wrong!" In my dream she was not an interlocutor but an adversary. How pathetic is it to dream what is obvious?

"I think she enjoyed being mean to you," her grandson tells me.

I have no doubt.

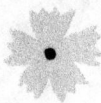

My insistence on asymmetries in this book should be careful not to ignore symmetries; the dancing pendulum of her life always crossed a stable center.

There were moments when Beverly appeared lost, not only depressed and defeated but nearly disintegrated. But mostly she was fully present; she possessed an aggressive presence, sitting there in full view, formidable. She intimidated the hell out of me. She delighted me. At times she wanted my approval. Illness only partially figures into her presence. *Health. Illness.* In the end I recognize it was not so much that she moved between these two states as that they were absorbed into one another. Dressing children for school while experiencing severe chest pains. Sink-ing deep into the cushions of her couch, skin ashen, eyes closed, telling me about a vacation she is planning to the casinos on the shore. These were moments not of contradiction but of fullness—not good, not bad, but a rich, deforming fullness.

And then there was her presence in my writing. Beverly watched me take notes for years. She knew words would carry on without her, or rather after her, beyond a particular moment. She said so. But she couldn't stand me reading what I'd written back to her. The past could stay in my writing, but the present had no room for it. I told her once that I had given up on sympathy, that sympathy was exhausting. I couldn't keep up with her day to day, couldn't follow her ups and downs closely enough to know my place within them. She laughed and grunted, "Tell me about it."

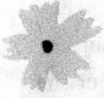

There is a purpose here, to conclude a decades-long

inquiry with a refusal to domesticate illness

and the sufferer for analytical expedience.

Even when nothing is recovered, no insight unearthed, nothing restored, and no final word given, we can say, knowing it is a falsehood, "That's all there is to say."

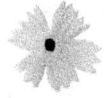

So, so, so in the absence of her I direct

my words at the hollow space of her.

Daily I remind myself: the future is not dependent on your

inability to describe your undoing.

LARA MIMOSA MONTES, *Thresholes*

REASSEMBLING

I was undone alongside Beverly, and she alongside me. Writing has been a way to record this double action of unraveling. What follows is a different, complementary action: a log of my resources as I attempted to repair what had been unmade—to reassemble scattered bits into something legible, through other people, through their works, words, wisdom, and encouragement.

THERE ARE STILL FINE PEOPLE in this world, people with enviable capacities for patience and generosity, intellectual or otherwise. I know a few of them. This work would not have been realized without the love and support of Fanny Gutiérrez-Meyers. I owe various debts of gratitude to Aude Bandini, Dominique Béhague, Cornelius Borck, David Caron, Stephen Chrisomalis, Thomas Cousins, Tarek Elhaik, Brian Goldstone, Talia Gordon, Jianbo Huang, Nancy Rose Hunt, Richard Keller, Junko Kitanaka, Abigail Lance–De Vos, Annette Leibing, Rhonda Lieber-man, Julie Livingston, Margaret Lock, Anne Lovell, Christos Lynteris, Kenneth MacLeish, Fiamma Montezemolo, Anand Pandian, Michelle Pentecost, Paul Rabinow, Eugene Raikhel, Jessica Robbins, and Vaibhav Saria. Richard Baxstrom and Stefanos Geroulanos are my intellectual companions, and their wisdom lines these pages. Conversations with Andrés Romero about his writing helped me with my own. Robert Des-jarlais and Anthony Stavrianakis have enriched and shaped my thinking. I am grateful to Ken Wissoker for his trust and enthusiasm. The book is dedicated to Pamela Reynolds, whose mentorship is a gift. While writing the book I moved from Baltimore to Detroit to Shanghai to Montréal. My colleagues along the way have been keenly supportive, for which I could not be more thankful.

There are people who listened and offered advice at different stages of my writing and thinking. At Emory University I thank Elissa Marder, Geoffrey Bennington, and Elizabeth Wilson; at Goldsmiths, thanks go to Marsha Rosengarten, Sophie Day, Monica Greco, Martin Savransky Duran, and Patricio Rojas Navarro; at a workshop hosted by the Fonda-tion Brocher in Geneva, Switzerland, I thank Lukas Engelmann, Janina Kehr, Fanny Chabrol, Gerald Oppenheimer, Christian McMillen, and Cindy Patton; at the Centre Marc Bloch, Berlin, and the Max-Planck-Institut für Wissenschaftsgeschichte, I am grateful to Sandra Laugier, Sabine Arnaud, Estelle Ferrarese, Penelope Deutscher, Daniele Loren-zini, Perig Pitrou, and John Carson for their encouragement. Thanks go to Céline Lefève, Claude-Olivier Doron, and Alexis Zimmer for orga-nizing an "Institut la personne en médecine" seminar in Paris. Vincent Gullin and Alexandra Bacopoulos-Viau generously invited me to present my work in the "Psy-ences" colloquia at the Centre interuniversitaire de recherché sur la science et la technologie at the Université du Québec à Montréal, and Junko Kitanaka created occasions for me to share ideas with her colleagues at Keio University, Tokyo, Japan. I found quiet moments to work on this material in the midst of other projects and commitments. I was a guest researcher at the Freiburg Institute for Advanced Studies (FRAIS)–Albert-Ludwigs-Universität Freiburg thanks to Nancy Campbell and Hermann Herlinghaus. I held a collaborative research fellowship with Stefanos Geroulanos from the American Council of Learned Societies and a residential research fellowship from the Eisenberg Institute for Historical Studies, University of Michigan.

My first effort to turn fieldwork into writing was a paper titled "La presence, le mourir et l'anthropologie du patient," which I presented at the Collège international de philosophie in Paris, France. Paola Marrati and François Roussel helped to set things in motion. I later published a paper titled "A Turn towards Dying: Presence, Signature, and the Social Course of Chronic Illness in Urban America" in *Medical Anthropology* 26, no. 3 (2007): 205–27. After I returned to Baltimore with hopes of reconciliation with Beverly, I published two essays: "How Is Comorbidity Lived?" in *Lancet* 386, no. 9999 (2015): 1128–29, and "The Poisonous Ingenuity of Time" in a special issue of *South Atlantic Quarterly* 115, no. 2 (2016): 351–65. I am grateful to Richard Keller and Sara Guyer for including me in their special issue and in the Sawyer Seminar on Biopolitics at the Humanities Center, University of Wisconsin–Madison, which resulted in lively discussions with Tim Campbell, Rob Mitchell, Jason E. Smith, and Donna Jones. Céline Lefève and Frédéric Worms invited me to publish a small book, *Chroniques de la maladie chronique* (2017), to expand previously published work and reflect on chronic illness and care, which was included in their "Questions de soin" collection at Presses Universitaires de France. Beverly is its subject, but *Chroniques* is a different book than this one. Even when I return to a few of the same moments, I do so from a less stable vantage point. The book here is a record of losing ground. After the publication of *Chroniques*, Céline and Frédéric organized a discussion at the École normale supérieure where

Claire Marin imparted superb insights and Jean-Christophe Weber's words intensified my commitment to return to Beverly in a different way (*m'a semblé très proche de ce que Barthes rapporte de Pasolini: une vitalité désespérée. Non pas la vitalité de la volonté de puissance, mais celle du désir de durer*). Anthony Stavrianakis and Nicolas Dodier invited me to present material at a workshop on "assemblages" at the École des hautes études en sciences sociales, which resulted in a paper titled "Lorsque le regard change: Singularité et modalités de l'image; *déclinaison en trois scènes*" for *Raisons pratiques* 28 (2018): 139–55, which appeared in English in a shorter form as "Trespass" in a forum on images in *Cultural Anthropology* organized by Aidan Seale-Feldman (Correspondences, *Fieldsights*, March 27, 2018, https://culanth.org/fieldsights/trespass). Finally, chapter 5, "A Living Room," appeared in a different form in the *History of Anthropology Newsletter* (February 4, 2019) thanks to the invitation of Cameron Brinitzer and Gabriel Coren.

In a different voice I thank Beverly's family. They have been inexplicably charitable with my intrusions on their lives. After years of phone calls and visits, followed by years of silence and my eventual return, they tolerated my questions and my preoccupations. They deserve more thanks than is possible to convey here.

Whatever this is, it started as research and then became something else. All names are pseudonyms. Beverly originally asked that I use her real name, but I was compelled to use a substitute. The irony is worth noting. One aim of this writing is to show the way Beverly secured meaning in illness and dying outside of institutions that might otherwise characterize that meaning for her. That, too, is not without limits.

NOTES

UNDOING

1. Todd Meyers and Nancy Rose Hunt, "The Other Global South," *Lancet* 384, no. 9958 (2014): 1921–22. In the essay we ask how a city like Detroit, which in so many ways reflects the concerns of other cities in the so-called global South, somehow sits uncomfortably within the logics of global humanitarianism and medical concern. We wrote about Detroit because we were in Detroit at the time, but Baltimore in its own way raises a similar set of questions, connected through histories of violence and inequality; see also Samuel Kelton Roberts Jr., *Infectious Fear: Politics, Disease, and the Health Effects of Segregation* (Chapel Hill: University of North Carolina Press, 2009); Thomas J. Sugrue, *The Origins of the Urban Crisis: Race and Inequality in Postwar Detroit* (Princeton, NJ: Princeton University Press, 1996); W. Michael Byrd and Linda A. Clayton, *An American Health Dilemma: A Medical History of African Americans and the Problem of Race, Beginnings to 1900* (New York: Routledge, 2000); Keith Wailoo, *Pain: A Political History* (Baltimore, MD: Johns Hopkins University Press, 2014); Harriet A. Washington, *Medical Apartheid: The Dark History of Medical Experimentation on Black Americans from Colonial Times to the Present* (New York: Doubleday, 2006); Alondra Nelson, *Body and Soul: The Black Panther Party and the Fight against Racial Discrimination* (Minneapolis: University of Minnesota Press, 2011); and Rana A. Hogarth, *Medicalizing Blackness: Making Racial Differences in the Atlantic World, 1780–1840* (Chapel Hill: University of North Carolina Press, 2017).

1. THESE MOMENTS FORMED BETWEEN US

1. Elizabeth A. Povinelli and Kim Turcot DiFruscia, "A Conversation with Elizabeth A. Povinelli," *Trans-Scripts* 2 (2012): 83; see also Elizabeth A. Povinelli, *Economies of Abandonment: Social Belonging and Endurance in Late Liberalism* (Durham, NC: Duke University Press, 2011).

2. Povinelli and DiFruscia, "Conversation with Elizabeth A. Povinelli," 83.

3. Stephen Best, *None like Us: Blackness, Belonging, Aesthetic Life* (Durham, NC: Duke University Press, 2019), 29.

4. Rachel R. Hardeman, Eduardo M. Medina, and Rhea W. Boyd, "Stolen Breaths," *New England Journal of Medicine* 383 (2020): 197–99; see also Dereck W. Paul Jr., Kelly R. Knight, Andre Campbell, and Louise Aronson, "Beyond a Moment—Reckoning with Our History and Embracing Antiracism in Medicine," *New England Journal of Medicine* 383 (2020): 1404–6.

5. Sara Ahmed, "Introduction," in Audre Lorde, *Your Silence Will Not Protect You* (London: Sliver, 2017), vi.

6. Audre Lorde, "Poetry Is Not a Luxury," in *The Master's Tools Will Never Dismantle the Master's House* (New York: Penguin Books, 2017), 1.

7. Christina Sharpe, *In the Wake: On Blackness and Being* (Durham, NC: Duke University Press, 2016), 134.

8. There are many examples of anthropological monographs centered on one individual: Lois Beck, *Nomad: A Year in the Life of a Qashqa'i Tribesman in Iran* (Berkeley: University of California Press, 1991); Unni Wikan, *Managing Turbulent Hearts: A Balinese Formula for Living* (Chicago: University of Chicago Press, 1990); João Biehl, *Vita: Life in a Zone of Social Abandonment* (Berkeley: University of California Press, 2013); Vincent Crapanzano, *Tuhami: Portrait of a Moroccan* (Chicago: University of Chicago Press, 1980); Mary F. Smith, *Baba of Karo: A Woman of the Muslim Hausa* (New York: Faber and Faber, 1954); and Marjorie Shostak, *Nisa: The Life and Words of a !Kung Woman* (London: Allen Lane, 1982). See also Jan Patrick Heiss, "Assessing Ernst Tugendhat's Philosophical Anthropology as a Theoretical Template for an Empirical Anthropology of the Individual," *Zeitschrift für Ethnologie* 140, no. 1 (2015): 35–54; and Jan Patrick Heiss and Albert Piette, "Individuals in Anthropology," *Zeitschrift für Ethnologie* 140, no. 1 (2015): 5–17. On the history of the use and scope of case studies, see John Forrester, *Thinking in Cases* (London: Polity, 2016).

9. I am thinking of three works in particular: Carlo Ginzburg, *Clues, Myths, and the Historical Method*, trans. John Tedeschi and Anne C. Tedeschi (Baltimore, MD: Johns Hopkins University Press, 2013); Carlo Ginzburg, *Threads and Traces: True False Fictive*, trans. Anne C. Tedeschi and John Tedeschi (Berkeley: University of California Press, 2012); and Paul Veyne, *Writing History: Essay on Epistemology*, trans. Mina Moore-Rinvolucri (Middletown, CT: Wesleyan University Press, 1984).

10. Michele K. Evans, Lisa Rosenbaum, Debra Malina, Stephen Morrissey, and Eric J. Rubin, "Diagnosing and Treating Systemic Racism," *New England Journal of Medicine* 383 (2020): 274–76; see also Clarence C. Gravlee and Elizabeth

Sweet, "Race, Ethnicity, and Racism in Medical Anthropology, 1977–2002," *Medical Anthropology Quarterly* 22, no. 1 (2008): 27–51; and David R. Williams, Jourdyn A. Lawrence, and Brigette A. Davis, "Racism and Health: Evidence and Needed Research," *Annual Review of Public Health* 40 (2019): 105–25.

11. John Hobersman, *Black and Blue: The Origins and Consequences of Medical Racism* (Berkeley: University of California Press, 2012).

12. Audre Lorde, "The Master's Tools Will Never Dismantle the Master's House," in *Your Silence Will Not Protect You* (London: Silver, 2017), 90.

2. STILL LIFE

1. Ian Hacking, *Representing and Intervening* (Cambridge: Cambridge University Press, 1983), 132. I am also thinking here of the passage from Ludwig Wittgenstein with which Elaine Scarry opens her book *On Beauty and Being Just* (Princeton, NJ: Princeton University Press, 2001): "What is the felt experience of cognition at the moment one stands in the presence of a beautiful boy or flower or bird? It seems to incite, even to require, the act of replication. Wittgenstein says that when the eye sees something beautiful, the hand wants to draw it" (3). But I might appreciate even more Jean-Luc Nancy's first line of *The Pleasure in Drawing*, trans. Philip Armstrong (New York: Fordham University Press, 2013): "Drawing is the opening of form" (1).

2. This thought is borrowed from Kathleen Stewart, *Ordinary Affects* (Durham, NC: Duke University Press, 2007), 7. The idea of "moving closer" in Stewart's work shares kinship with Theodor Adorno's thoughts on Walter Benjamin's writing by way of method: "The thoughts press close to its objects, seek to touch it, smell it, taste it and thereby transform itself." Theodor Adorno, *Prisms* (Cambridge, MA: MIT Press, 1983), 240; see also Walter Benjamin, *The Arcades Project*, trans. Howard Eiland and Kevin McLaughlin (Cambridge, MA: Harvard University Press, 1999); and Lauren Berlant, "Slow Death (Sovereignty, Obesity, Lateral Agency)," *Critical Inquiry* 33, no. 4 (2007): 754–80.

3. John Berger, *Bento's Sketchbook* (New York: Pantheon, 2011), 44.

4. Berger, *Bento's Sketchbook*, 106.

5. Berger, *Bento's Sketchbook*, 35–37.

6. Susan Stewart, *On Longing* (Durham, NC: Duke University Press, 1992), 13.

7. Two thinkers immediately come to mind: Tarek Elhaik talks about a "zone of mutual intrusion" in his *The Incurable Image* (Edinburgh: University of Edinburgh Press, 2016), and Maggie Nelson welcomes contamination as a quality of our relationships as they become intimate in *The Argonauts* (Minneapolis: Graywolf, 2015) and considers the possibility of rupture as a quality of care in *The Art*

of Cruelty (New York: Norton, 2011). It is also impossible not to loop in and out of the thought of Paul Rabinow, especially in *The Accompaniment: Assembling the Contemporary* (Chicago: University of Chicago Press, 2011).

3. THE ACCIDENT OF CONTACT

1. W. G. Sebald, *The Rings of Saturn*, trans. Michael Hulse (New York: New Directions, 2016), 212.

2. Berger, *Bento's Sketchbook*, 23.

4. RESUSCITATIONS

1. Anand Pandian, *Ayya's Accounts: A Ledger of Hope in Modern India* (Bloomington: Indiana University Press, 2014). I return often to Pandian's *Crooked Stalks: Cultivating Virtue in South India* (Durham, NC: Duke University Press, 2009).

2. Care is indeed a conundrum. I have abandoned any attempt to unify a picture of care, of what it is, what it represents, and its actions—it is an understatement to say that I have lost my urge to resolve conflicting theories or temperaments. I am thinking here with the words of Christina Crosby, from her memoir, *A Body, Undone: Living On after Great Pain* (New York: New York University Press, 2016): "I know for sure that we are much more profoundly interdependent creatures than we often care to think; and I know imperatively that we need a calculus that can value caring labor far differently than we do today" (4). I am most concerned, here in my moments with Beverly, with the question, "Can I call this care *or are there other terms for what is happening*?" Crucially, what conditions attach themselves to these terms, what are their substance and their flesh, and what do I do with concepts when actions stretch relationships thin or when they contract or pinch? (My thinking here is aided by the forthcoming writing of Andrés Romero, from his work in Bogotá, Colombia, which I find key to addressing these questions.) This is an incomplete list, but I am thinking care in at least three streams: The first is the work of anthropologists including (especially) Lisa Stevenson, *Life beside Itself: Imagining Care in the Canadian Arctic* (Berkeley: University of California Press, 2014), João Biehl, *Will to Live: AIDS Therapies and the Politics of Survival* (Princeton, NJ: Princeton University Press, 2007), and Pamela Reynolds, *War in Worcester: Youth and the Apartheid State* (New York: Fordham University Press, 2012)—ethnographic works that are historically aware and relationally nuanced. The second stream is the writings of French thinkers inside and outside of medical environments that consider how the act of offering

care as intervention exposes the character of expectations held by others—scholarship concerned with the ways philosophies of care, either explicitly or assumed, are enacted, especially the work of Céline Lefève (see her book series at Presses Universitaires de France with Frédéric Worms, "Questions de soin," and a number of other collections: Céline Lefève, Jean-Christophe Mino, and Nathalie Zaccaï-Reyners, *Le soin: Approches contemporaines* [Paris: Presses Universitaires de France, 2016]; Lazare Benaroyo, Céline Lefève, Jean-Christophe Mino, and Frédéric Worms, *La philosophie du soin: Éthique, médecine, et société* [Paris: Presses Universitaires de France, 2010]; Céline Lefève, Lazare Benaroyo, and Frédéric Worms, eds., *Les classiques du soin* [Paris: Presses Universitaires de France, 2015]); included here is the psychoanalytically informed humanism of Cynthia Fleury, *Le soin est un humanism* (Paris: Gallimard, 2019), and the projects of Sandra Laugier, through the thought of Stanley Cavell, which also facilitates a return to feminist scholars, most especially Carol Gilligan. The third stream is scholarship that pulls the domestic into the context of medicine, including work by anthropologists such as Annette Leibing (see, for example, "Fallacies of Care: When Meaning Well Does Harm," in her coedited special section in *Journal of Aging Studies* 51 [2019]: 1–10); Sameena Mulla (*Violence and Care: Rape Victims, Forensic Nurses, and Sexual Assault Intervention* [New York: New York University Press, 2014]); Zoë Wool (on injury and grief, see her "Mourning, Affect, Sociality: On the Possibilities of Open Grief," *Cultural Anthropology* 35, no. 1 [2020]: 40–47); Anne M. Lovell (see her "Debating Life after Disaster: Charity Hospital Babies and Bioscientific Futures in Post-Katrina New Orleans," *Medical Anthropology Quarterly* 25 [2011]: 254–77); Janelle S. Taylor ("On Recognition, Caring, and Dementia," *Medical Anthropology Quarterly* 22 [2008]: 313–35); and Arthur Kleinman ("Varieties of Experiences of Care," *Perspectives in Biology and Medicine* 63, no. 3 [2020]: 458–65).

3. Sharpe, *In the Wake*, 134.

4. Lived, not prescribed. I feel unease using terms like *everyday ethics* or *ordinary ethics*—terms popularized in the writing of Veena Das, Michael Lambek, Webb Keane, Didier Fassin, and others (see Lambek et al., *Four Lectures on Ethics: Anthropological Perspectives* [Chicago: HAU, 2015]). I worry that the locus of this reading of ethics might sit adjacent to the individual. I worry its pitch might drown out shakier voices, and that invention (or surprise, or conflict) is outpaced by prescription. Finally, I worry about the danger of an ethics that is already in mind and that somehow finds agreement from the outset.

5. A LIVING ROOM

This chapter appeared in a different form in the *History of Anthropology Newsletter* (February 4, 2019).

1. John Berger, "Means to Live," in *Understanding a Photograph*, ed. Geoff Dyer (New York: Aperture, 2013), 108–10.

2. Berger, "Means to Live," 109.

3. Todd Meyers, *The Clinic and Elsewhere* (Seattle: University of Washington Press, 2013).

4. Georges Canguilhem, "Le vivant et son milieu," in *La connaissance de la vie* (Paris: Vrin, 1952), 165–98; translated as "The Living and Its Milieu," in *Knowledge of Life*, ed. Paola Marrati and Todd Meyers, trans. Stefanos Geroulanos and Daniela Ginsburg (New York: Fordham University Press, 2008), 98–120.

5. François Dagognet, *Le corps* (Paris: Presses Universitaires de France, 2008).

6. Kurt Goldstein, *The Organism* (New York: Zone Books, 1995).

7. Canguilhem, "Living and Its Milieu," 102–4.

8. Canguilhem, "Living and Its Milieu," 113.

9. Canguilhem, "Living and Its Milieu," 117.

6. THOUGHTS OF SUICIDE

Preceding epigraph: As an alternative quote that punctuates horror and banality, I think of John Berger's "Born 05/11/26" (1983):

> no more thoughts of suicide
>> than is normal in November

The quote is found in *Soundings* 58 (2014): 101. I am also thinking here of *The Seasons in Quincy: Four Portraits of John Berger* (dir. Bartek Dziadosz, Colin MacCabe, Christopher Roth, and Tilda Swinton, 2016), which highlights his experiments in openness so near the end.

1. On the final gesture, see Anthony Stavrianakis's brilliant and challenging *Leaving: A Narrative of Assisted Suicide* (Berkeley: University of California Press, 2020), a book that is a resource for both its tone and its ability to demonstrate how thought is tested.

7. [. . .]

Preceding epigraph: Hiroshi Sugimoto, *Seascapes* (New York: Damiani Editore, 2015), n.p.:

Water and air. So very commonplace are these substances, they hardly attract attention—and yet they vouchsafe our very existence. The beginnings of life are shrouded in myth: Let there water and air. Living phenomena spontaneously generated from water and air in the presence of light, though that could just as easily suggest random coincidence as a Deity. Let's just say that there happened to be a planet with water and air in our solar system, and moreover at precisely the right distance from the sun for the temperatures required to coax forth life. While hardly inconceivable that at least one such planet should exist in the vast reaches of universe, we search in vain for another similar example. Mystery of mysteries, water and air are right there before us in the sea. Every time I view the sea, I feel a calming sense of security, as if visiting my ancestral home; I embark on a voyage of seeing.

1. Roland Barthes, *Camera Lucida: Reflections on Photography*, trans. Richard Howard (New York: Hill and Wang, 1981), 27: "*Punctum* is also: sting, speck, cut, little hole—and also a cast of the dice. A photograph's *punctum* is that accident which pricks me (but also bruises me, is poignant to me)."

2. Dan Fox, *Limbo* (London: Fitzcarraldo Editions, 2018), 69.

8. BREATHING FEELS LIKE A FALSEHOOD

Preceding epigraph: See also Stefanie Heine's incredible essay on the rhythm of breathing and pauses in writing: "'animi velut respirant': Rhythm and Breathing Pauses in Ancient Rhetoric, Virginia Woolf, and Robert Musil," *Comparative Literature* 69, no. 4 (2017): 355–69.

1. On a body maimed, see Julietta Singh's powerful *No Archive Will Restore You* (Goleta, CA: Punctum Books, 2018).

2. On the troubled politics of breathing, Frantz Fanon borrows words from the poet Aimé Césaire's *Cahier d'un retour au pays natal* (Paris: Présence Africaine, 1956), 78; see Frantz Fanon, *Black Skin, White Masks*, trans. Charles Lam Markmann (New York: Grove, 1967), 124–25:

But they abandon themselves, possessed, to the essence
of all things, knowing nothing of externals but possessed by the movement
of all things.

uncaring to subdue but playing the play of the world
truly the eldest sons of the world
open to all the breaths of the world
meeting-place of all the winds of the world
undrained bed of all the waters of the world

spark of the sacred fire of the World
flesh of the flesh of the world, throbbing with the
very movement of the world!

For Césaire, respiration—the breath, the action of breathing—carries life and its possibility. He insists on the double action of vitalism and world-making; breathing is a way of moving into and within new worlds.

3. Thomas Mann, *The Magic Mountain*, trans. H. T. Lowe-Porter (New York: Alfred A. Knopf, 1930), 352, 362–63.

4. Michel Foucault, *The Birth of the Clinic*, trans. A. M. Sheridan (New York: Vintage, 1973), 153; see also Georges Canguilhem, *Writings on Medicine*, trans. Stefanos Geroulanos and Todd Meyers (New York: Fordham University Press, 2012).

5. Mann, *Magic Mountain*, 373; Virginia Woolf, *On Being Ill* (1930; Ashfield, MA: Paris Press, 2002), 12.

9. NOTES ON A NEW MORALISM

1. Thomas Bernhard, *Woodcutters*, trans. David McLintock (New York: Vintage International, 2010); see also *Gathering Evidence and My Prizes: A Memoir*, trans. David McLintock (New York: Vintage International, 2011).

2. Osamu Dazai, *No Longer Human*, trans. Donald Keene (New York: New Directions, 1973).

3. Georges Canguilhem, "Health: Popular Concept and Philosophical Question," in *Writings on Medicine*, 43–52.

4. Canguilhem, "Health," 44.

5. I discuss this quote by Michaux in an essay titled "Mastery and Its Opposite: Learning at Art School with Rhonda Lieberman," in *The Rhonda Lieberman Reader*, ed. Sarah Lehrer-Graiwer (Los Angeles: Pep Talk Reader, 2018), 491–95.

6. Karl Ove Knausgaard, *My Struggle, Book 1*, trans. Don Bartlett (New York: Farrar, Straus and Giroux, 2013), 9.

7. It is hard to name precisely what it is that is so poignant when Beverly is thrust into the middle of the phantastical. I am convinced that clues can be found in the writing of Toni Morrison; as Vanessa D. Dickerson writes so perceptively of Morrison's characters, they are freed from the reduction of their representation when they enter "a liminal space such as illness or the otherworldly." See Vanessa D. Dickerson, "Summoning SomeBody: The Flesh Made Word in Toni Morrison's Fiction," in *Recovering the Black Female Body*, ed. Michael Bennett and Vanessa D. Dickerson (Piscataway, NJ: Rutgers University Press, 2000), 196.

8. Erin Manning, *For a Pragmatics of the Useless* (Durham, NC: Duke University Press, 2020).

9. See a quote by Maurice Merleau-Ponty in Stefanos Geroulanos's *An Atheism That Is Not Humanist Emerges in French Thought*: "to disassociate from the idea of a humanity fully guaranteed by natural law and not only reconcile consciousness of human values and consciousness of the infrastructures which keep them in existence, but insist upon their inseparability." Maurice Merleau-Ponty, "Man and Adversity," in *Signs*, trans. Richard C. McCleary (Evanston, IL: Northwestern University Press, 1964), 232–35; in Stefanos Geroulanos, *An Atheism That Is Not Humanist Emerges in French Thought* (Palo Alto, CA: Stanford University Press, 2010), 15.

10. On a "negative philosophical anthropology," see Geroulanos, *An Atheism That Is Not Humanist*, 48–51, 174–77, and 194–199; Emmanuel Lévinas, *On Escape*, trans. Bettina Bergo (Palo Alto, CA: Stanford University Press, 2003), and *Humanism of the Other*, trans. Nidra Poller (Chicago: University of Illinois Press, 2003); and Lévinas's essay on Maurice Blanchot, "The Poet's Vision," in *Proper Names*, trans. Michael Smith (Palo Alto, CA: Stanford University Press, 1996), 127–39. For an important discussion of Geroulanos's *An Atheism That Is Not Humanist Emerges in French Thought*, see Stefanos Geroulanos, "Secularism, Atheism, Antihumanism," *The Immanent Frame*, Social Science Research Council (SSRC), June 3, 2010, https://tif.ssrc.org/2010/06/03/secularism-atheism-antihumanism/.

11. Cheryl Mattingly, *Moral Laboratories: Family Peril and the Struggle for a Good Life* (Berkeley: University of California Press, 2014).

12. See especially Zakiyyah Iman Jackson's spectacular *Becoming Human: Matter and Meaning in an Antiblack World* (New York: New York University Press, 2020).

13. I am awed by the insights of Lisa Stevenson in "Looking Away," *Cultural Anthropology* 35, no. 1 (2020): 6–13.

14. Woolf, *On Being Ill*, 11.

15. I am thinking here of technologies of truth in Michel Foucault's *The History of Sexuality*, vol. 1, *An Introduction*, trans. Robert Hurley (New York: Random House, 1978); the section on the cultivation of the self in *The History of Sexuality*, vol. 3, *The Care of the Self*, trans. Robert Hurley (New York: Random House, 1986); and a wholly different mode of confession in *The History of Sexuality*, vol. 4, *Confessions of the Flesh*, trans. Robert Hurley (New York: Pantheon, 2021).

16. For an analysis that puts Michel Foucault and Frantz Fanon into conversation around the question of confession, see Daniele Lorenzini and Martina Tazzioli, "Confessional Subjects and Conducts of Non-truth: Foucault, Fanon, and the Making of the Subject," *Theory, Culture and Society* 35, no. 1 (2018): 71–90.

17. Anne Boyer, *The Undying: Pain, Vulnerability, Mortality, Medicine, Art, Time, Dreams, Data, Exhaustion, Cancer, and Care* (New York: Farrar, Straus and Giroux, 2019), 252.

10. BLACK FIGURINE

1. Michael Taussig, *Mimesis and Alterity: A Particular History of the Senses* (New York: Routledge, 1993), 14; see also Paul Stoller, *Embodying Colonial Memories* (New York: Routledge, 1995).

2. Taussig, *Mimesis and Alterity*, 14.

3. William Pietz, "The Problem of the Fetish," *Res*, no. 9 (1986): 5–17; see also Fred R. Myers, "Introduction: The Empire of Things," in *The Empire of Things: Regimes of Value and Material Culture*, ed. Fred R. Meyers (Santa Fe: School of American Research Press, 2001), 3–62; and Rosalind C. Morris, "'Fetishism (Supposing That It Existed)': A Preface to the Translation of Charles de Brosses's Transgression," in *The Return of Fetishism: Charles de Brosses and the Afterlives of an Idea*, ed. Rosalind C. Morris and Daniel H. Leonard (Chicago: University of Chicago Press, 2017), vii–xvi.

4. Berger, *Bento's Sketchbook*, 37.

5. Joan Didion, *The Year of Magical Thinking* (New York: Knopf, 2005).

6. Robert Desjarlais, *The Blind Man: A Phantasmography* (New York: Fordham University Press, 2018).

7. Michael Taussig, *Mastery of Non-mastery in the Age of Meltdown* (Chicago: University of Chicago Press, 2020); see also Meyers, "Mastery and Its Opposite."

8. Roland Barthes, *Mourning Diary*, trans. Richard Howard (New York: Hill and Wang, 2012), 6, 7.

9. Roland Barthes, *The Neutral*, trans. Rosalind Krauss and Denis Hollier (New York: Columbia University Press, 2007), xiii, 6. See Anthony Stavrianakis's discussion in *Leaving*; see also Desjarlais, *Blind Man*—I find Desjarlais's phantasmography endlessly instructive, specifically his commitment to the phantasm as a method:

> "Phantasm" is considered here in the variable sense of an apparition or illusions; a ghost or phantom; an imaginary construct; a fantastical image or vision; a haunting memory; a fanciful idea; or a cohering fantasy, momentary or lifelong, conscious or unconscious. This book, then, is a compendium of phantasms. To paraphrase one passage, so much in life is imagined, not concretely real, and an anthropology attuned to the imaginary—a fantastical anthropology, an anthropology of the phantasmal—needs to account for the force and tenor of the imagined, the possible, the conjectured,

the feared and dreamed of, specters of memory and perception, within the phantasmal flow of its thought and expression. (ix)

I return to the passage as a confirmation of possibility. One last point of contact on correspondence with the dead: see Vinciane Despret, *Au bonheur des morts* (Paris: Le Découverte, 2015).

10. Barthes, *Neutral*, 10.

11. Barthes, *Neutral*, 11.

12. Roland Barthes, *The Responsibility of Forms*, trans. Richard Howard (New York: Hill and Wang, 1985), 160.

13. William Kentridge and Rosalind C. Morris, *That Which Is Not Drawn* (London: Seagull Books, 2014).

14. Barthes, *Responsibility of Forms*, 165.

BIBLIOGRAPHY

Adorno, Theodor. *Prisms*. Cambridge, MA: MIT Press, 1983.

Ahmed, Sara. "Introduction." In Audre Lorde, *Your Silence Will Not Protect You*, v–xii. London: Sliver, 2017.

Bachelard, Gaston. *The Poetics of Space*. Translated by Maria Jolas. 1958. New York: Penguin Books, 2014.

Barthes, Roland. *Camera Lucida: Reflections on Photography*. Translated by Richard Howard. New York: Hill and Wang, 1981.

Barthes, Roland. *Mourning Diary*. Translated by Richard Howard. New York: Hill and Wang, 2012.

Barthes, Roland. *The Neutral*. Translated by Rosalind Krauss and Denis Hollier. New York: Columbia University Press, 2007.

Barthes, Roland. *The Responsibility of Forms*. Translated by Richard Howard. New York: Hill and Wang, 1985.

Beck, Lois. *Nomad: A Year in the Life of a Qashqa'i Tribesman in Iran*. Berkeley: University of California Press, 1991.

Benaroyo, Lazare, Céline Lefève, Jean-Christophe Mino, and Frédéric Worms. *La philosophie du soin: Éthique, médecine, et société*. Paris: Presses Universitaires de France, 2010.

Benjamin, Walter. *The Arcades Project*. Translated by Howard Eiland and Kevin McLaughlin. Cambridge, MA: Harvard University Press, 1999.

Berger, John. *Bento's Sketchbook*. New York: Pantheon, 2011.

Berger, John. "Born 05/11/26." 1983. *Soundings* 58 (2014): 101.

Berger, John. "The Hour of Poetry." 1982. In *Selected Essays*, edited by Geoff Dyer, 445–52. New York: Vintage, 2003.

Berger, John. "Means to Live." In *Understanding a Photograph*, edited and introduced by Geoff Dyer, 108–10. New York: Aperture, 2013.

Berlant, Lauren. "Slow Death (Sovereignty, Obesity, Lateral Agency)." *Critical Inquiry* 33, no. 4 (2007): 754–80.

Bernhard, Thomas. *Gathering Evidence and My Prizes: A Memoir*. Translated by David McLintock. New York: Vintage International, 2011.

Bernhard, Thomas. *The Loser*. Translated by Jack Dawson. New York: Random House, 1991.

Bernhard, Thomas. *Woodcutters*. Translated by David McLintock. New York: Vintage International, 2010.

Best, Stephen. *None like Us: Blackness, Belonging, Aesthetic Life*. Durham, NC: Duke University Press, 2019.

Biehl, João. *Vita: Life in a Zone of Social Abandonment*. Berkeley: University of California Press, 2013.

Biehl, João. *Will to Live: AIDS Therapies and the Politics of Survival*. Princeton, NJ: Princeton University Press, 2007.

Boyer, Anne. *The Undying: Pain, Vulnerability, Mortality, Medicine, Art, Time, Dreams, Data, Exhaustion, Cancer, and Care*. New York: Farrar, Straus and Giroux, 2019.

Byrd, W. Michael, and Linda A. Clayton. *An American Health Dilemma: A Medical History of African Americans and the Problem of Race, Beginnings to 1900*. New York: Routledge, 2000.

Canguilhem, Georges. "The Living and Its Milieu." In *Knowledge of Life*, edited by Paola Marrati and Todd Meyers, translated by Stefanos Geroulanos and Daniela Ginsburg, 98–120. New York: Fordham University Press, 2008. Originally published as "Le vivant et son milieu," in *La connaissance de la vie*, 165–98 (Paris: Vrin, 1952).

Canguilhem, Georges. *Writings on Medicine*. Translated by Stefanos Geroulanos and Todd Meyers. New York: Fordham University Press, 2012.

Césaire, Aimé. *Cahier d'un retour au pays natal*. Paris: Présence Africaine, 1956.

Crapanzano, Vincent. *Tuhamti: Portrait of a Moroccan*. Chicago: University of Chicago Press, 1980.

Crosby, Christina. *A Body, Undone: Living On after Great Pain*. New York: New York University Press, 2016.

Dagognet, François. *Le corps*. Paris: Presses Universitaires de France, 2008.

Dazai, Osamu. *No Longer Human*. Translated by Donald Keene. New York: New Directions, 1973.

Desjarlais, Robert. *The Blind Man: A Phantasmography*. New York: Fordham University Press, 2018.

Despret, Vinciane. *Au bonheur des morts*. Paris: Le Découverte, 2015.

Dickerson, Vanessa D. "Summoning SomeBody: The Flesh Made Word in Toni Morrison's Fiction." In *Recovering the Black Female Body*, edited by

Michael Bennett and Vanessa D. Dickerson, 195–216. Piscataway, NJ: Rutgers University Press, 2000.

Didion, Joan. *The Year of Magical Thinking.* New York: Knopf, 2005.

Elhaik, Tarek. *The Incurable Image.* Edinburgh: University of Edinburgh Press, 2016.

Evans, Michele K., Lisa Rosenbaum, Debra Malina, Stephen Morrissey, and Eric J. Rubin. "Diagnosing and Treating Systemic Racism." *New England Journal of Medicine* 383 (2020): 274–76.

Fanon, Frantz. *Black Skin, White Masks.* Translated by Charles Lam Markmann. New York: Grove, 1967.

Fleury, Cynthia. *Le soin est un humanism.* Paris: Gallimard, 2019.

Forrester, John. *Thinking in Cases.* London: Polity, 2016.

Foucault, Michel. *The Birth of the Clinic.* Translated by A. M. Sheridan. New York: Vintage, 1973.

Foucault, Michel. *The History of Sexuality.* Vol. 1, *An Introduction.* Translated by Robert Hurley. New York: Random House, 1978.

Foucault, Michel. *The History of Sexuality.* Vol. 3, *The Care of the Self.* Translated by Robert Hurley. New York: Random House, 1986.

Foucault, Michel. *The History of Sexuality.* Vol. 4, *Confessions of the Flesh.* Translated by Robert Hurley. New York: Pantheon, 2021.

Fox, Dan. *Limbo.* London: Fitzcarraldo Editions, 2018.

Geroulanos, Stefanos. *An Atheism That Is Not Humanist Emerges in French Thought.* Palo Alto, CA: Stanford University Press, 2010.

Geroulanos, Stefanos. "Secularism, Atheism, Antihumanism." *The Immanent Frame,* Social Science Research Council (SSRC), June 3, 2010. https://tif.ssrc .org/2010/06/03/secularism-atheism-antihumanism/.

Ginzburg, Carlo. *Clues, Myths, and the Historical Method.* Translated by John Tedeschi and Anne C. Tedeschi. Baltimore, MD: Johns Hopkins University Press, 2013.

Ginzburg, Carlo. *Threads and Traces: True False Fictive.* Translated by Anne C. Tedeschi and John Tedeschi. Berkeley: University of California Press, 2012.

Goldstein, Kurt. *The Organism.* New York: Zone Books, 1995.

Gravlee, Clarence C., and Elizabeth Sweet. "Race, Ethnicity, and Racism in Medical Anthropology, 1977–2002." *Medical Anthropology Quarterly* 22, no. 1 (2008): 27–51.

Hacking, Ian. *Representing and Intervening.* Cambridge: Cambridge University Press, 1983.

Hardeman, Rachel R., Eduardo M. Medina, and Rhea W. Boyd. "Stolen Breaths." *New England Journal of Medicine* 383 (2020): 197–99.

Heine, Stefanie. "'animi velut respirant': Rhythm and Breathing Pauses in Ancient Rhetoric, Virginia Woolf, and Robert Musil." *Comparative Literature* 69, no. 4 (2017): 355–69.

Heiss, Jan Patrick. "Assessing Ernst Tugendhat's Philosophical Anthropology as a Theoretical Template for an Empirical Anthropology of the Individual." *Zeitschrift für Ethnologie* 140, no. 1 (2015): 35–54.

Heiss, Jan Patrick, and Albert Piette. "Individuals in Anthropology." *Zeitschrift für Ethnologie* 140 (2015): 5–17.

Hobersman, John. *Black and Blue: The Origins and Consequences of Medical Racism*. Berkeley: University of California Press, 2012.

Hogarth, Rana A. *Medicalizing Blackness: Making Racial Differences in the Atlantic World, 1780–1840*. Chapel Hill: University of North Carolina Press, 2017.

Jackson, Zakiyyah Iman. *Becoming Human: Matter and Meaning in an Antiblack World*. New York: New York University Press, 2020.

Kentridge, William, and Rosalind C. Morris. *That Which Is Not Drawn*. London: Seagull Books, 2014.

Kleinman, Arthur. "Varieties of Experiences of Care." *Perspectives in Biology and Medicine* 63 (2020): 458–65.

Knausgaard, Karl Ove. *My Struggle, Book 1*. Translated by Don Bartlett. New York: Farrar, Straus and Giroux, 2013.

Lambek, Michael, Veena Das, Didier Fassin, and Webb Keane. *Four Lectures on Ethics: Anthropological Perspectives*. Chicago: HAU, 2015.

Lefève, Céline, Lazare Benaroyo, and Frédéric Worms, eds. *Les classiques du soin*. Paris: Presses Universitaires de France, 2015.

Lefève, Céline, Jean-Christophe Mino, and Nathalie Zaccaï-Reyners. *Le soin: Approches contemporaines*. Paris: Presses Universitaires de France, 2016.

Leibing, Annette. "Fallacies of Care: When Meaning Well Does Harm." *Journal of Aging Studies* 51 (2019): 1–10.

Lévinas, Emmanuel. *Humanism of the Other*. Translated by Nidra Poller. Chicago: University of Illinois Press, 2003.

Lévinas, Emmanuel. *On Escape*. Translated by Bettina Bergo. Palo Alto, CA: Stanford University Press, 2003.

Lévinas, Emmanuel. *Proper Names*. Translated by Michael Smith. Palo Alto, CA: Stanford University Press, 1996.

Lorde, Audre. *The Master's Tools Will Never Dismantle the Master's House*. New York: Penguin Books, 2017.

Lorde, Audre. *Your Silence Will Not Protect You*. London: Sliver, 2017.

Lorenzini, Daniele, and Martina Tazzioli. "Confessional Subjects and Conducts of Non-truth: Foucault, Fanon, and the Making of the Subject." *Theory, Culture and Society* 35, no. 1 (2018): 71–90.

Lovell, Anne M. "Debating Life after Disaster: Charity Hospital Babies and Bioscientific Futures in Post-Katrina New Orleans." *Medical Anthropology Quarterly* 25, no. 2 (2011): 254–77.

Mann, Thomas. *The Magic Mountain*. Translated by H. T. Lowe-Porter. New York: Alfred A. Knopf, 1930.

Manning, Erin. *For a Pragmatics of the Useless*. Durham, NC: Duke University Press, 2020.

Mattingly, Cheryl. *Moral Laboratories: Family Peril and the Struggle for a Good Life*. Berkeley: University of California Press, 2014.

Merleau-Ponty, Maurice. "Man and Adversity." In *Signs*, translated by Richard C. McCleary, 232–35. Evanston, IL: Northwestern University Press, 1964.

Meyers, Todd. *The Clinic and Elsewhere*. Seattle: University of Washington Press, 2013.

Meyers, Todd. "Mastery and Its Opposite: Learning at Art School with Rhonda Lieberman." In *The Rhonda Lieberman Reader*, edited by Sarah Lehrer-Graiwer, 491–95. Los Angeles: Pep Talk Reader, 2018.

Meyers, Todd, and Nancy Rose Hunt. "The Other Global South." *Lancet* 384, no. 9958 (2014): 1921–22.

Montes, Lara Mimosa. *Thresholes*. Minneapolis: Coffee House, 2020.

Morris, Rosalind C. "'Fetishism (Supposing That It Existed)': A Preface to the Translation of Charles de Brosses's Transgression." In Charles de Brosses, Rosalind C. Morris, and Daniel H. Leonard, *The Return of Fetishism: Charles de Brosses and the Afterlives of an Idea*, vii–xvi. Chicago: University of Chicago Press, 2017.

Mulla, Sameena. *Violence and Care: Rape Victims, Forensic Nurses, and Sexual Assault Intervention*. New York: New York University Press, 2014.

Myers, Fred R. "Introduction: The Empire of Things." In *The Empire of Things: Regimes of Value and Material Culture*, edited by Fred R. Myers, 3–62. Santa Fe: School of American Research Press, 2001.

Nancy, Jean-Luc. *The Pleasure in Drawing*. Translated by Philip Armstrong. New York: Fordham University Press, 2013.

Nelson, Alondra. *Body and Soul: The Black Panther Party and the Fight against Racial Discrimination*. Minneapolis: University of Minnesota Press, 2011.

Nelson, Maggie. *The Argonauts*. Minneapolis: Graywolf, 2015.

Nelson, Maggie. *The Art of Cruelty*. New York: Norton, 2011.

Nietzsche, Friedrich. *Thus Spoke Zarathustra*. In *The Portable Nietzsche*, edited and translated by Walter Kaufmann. New York: Penguin Books, 1954.

Pandian, Anand. *Ayya's Accounts: A Ledger of Hope in Modern India.* Bloomington: Indiana University Press, 2014.

Pandian, Anand. *Crooked Stalks: Cultivating Virtue in South India.* Durham, NC: Duke University Press, 2009.

Paul, Dereck W., Jr., Kelly R. Knight, Andre Campbell, and Louise Aronson. "Beyond a Moment—Reckoning with Our History and Embracing Antiracism in Medicine." *New England Journal of Medicine* 383 (2020): 1404–6.

Pietz, William. "The Problem of the Fetish." *Res*, no. 9 (1986): 5–17.

Povinelli, Elizabeth A. *Economies of Abandonment: Social Belonging and Endurance in Late Liberalism.* Durham, NC: Duke University Press, 2011.

Povinelli, Elizabeth A., and Kim Turcot DiFruscia. "A Conversation with Elizabeth A. Povinelli." *Trans-Scripts* 2 (2012): 76–90.

Rabinow, Paul. *The Accompaniment: Assembling the Contemporary.* Chicago: University of Chicago Press, 2011.

Reynolds, Pamela. *War in Worcester: Youth and the Apartheid State.* New York: Fordham University Press, 2012.

Riley, Denise. *Time Lived, without Its Flow.* London: Picador, 2019.

Roberts, Samuel Kelton, Jr. *Infectious Fear: Politics, Disease, and the Health Effects of Segregation.* Chapel Hill: University of North Carolina Press, 2009.

Scarry, Elaine. *On Beauty and Being Just.* Princeton, NJ: Princeton University Press, 2001.

Sebald, W. G. *The Rings of Saturn.* Translated by Michael Hulse. New York: New Directions, 2016.

Sharpe, Christina. *In the Wake: On Blackness and Being.* Durham, NC: Duke University Press, 2016.

Shostak, Marjorie. *Nisa: The Life and Words of a !Kung Woman.* London: Allen Lane, 1982.

Sinclair, Safiya. "In Childhood, Certain Skies Refined My Seeing." In *Cannibal*, 6–7. Lincoln: University of Nebraska Press, 2016.

Singh, Julietta. *No Archive Will Restore You.* Goleta, CA: Punctum Books, 2018.

Smith, Mary F. *Baba of Karo: A Woman of the Muslim Hausa.* New York: Faber and Faber, 1954.

Stavrianakis, Anthony. *Leaving: A Narrative of Assisted Suicide.* Berkeley: University of California Press, 2020.

Stevenson, Lisa. *Life beside Itself: Imagining Care in the Canadian Arctic.* Berkeley: University of California Press, 2014.

Stevenson, Lisa. "Looking Away." *Cultural Anthropology* 35, no. 1 (2020): 6–13.

Stewart, Kathleen. *Ordinary Affects.* Durham, NC: Duke University Press, 2007.

Stewart, Susan. *On Longing*. Durham, NC: Duke University Press, 1992.

Stoller, Paul. *Embodying Colonial Memories*. New York: Routledge, 1995.

Sugimoto, Hiroshi. *Seascapes*. New York: Damiani Editore, 2015.

Sugrue, Thomas J. *The Origins of the Urban Crisis: Race and Inequality in Postwar Detroit*. Princeton, NJ: Princeton University Press, 1996.

Taussig, Michael. *Mastery of Non-mastery in the Age of Meltdown*. Chicago: University of Chicago Press, 2020.

Taussig, Michael. *Mimesis and Alterity: A Particular History of the Senses*. New York: Routledge, 1993.

Taylor, Janelle S. "On Recognition, Caring, and Dementia." *Medical Anthropology Quarterly* 22, no. 4 (2008): 313–35.

Veyne, Paul. *Writing History: Essay on Epistemology*. Translated by Mina Moore-Rinvolucri. Middletown, CT: Wesleyan University Press, 1984.

Wailoo, Keith. *Pain: A Political History*. Baltimore, MD: Johns Hopkins University Press, 2014.

Washington, Harriet A. *Medical Apartheid: The Dark History of Medical Experimentation on Black Americans from Colonial Times to the Present*. New York: Doubleday, 2006.

Wikan, Unni. *Managing Turbulent Hearts: A Balinese Formula for Living*. Chicago: University of Chicago Press, 1990.

Williams, David R., Jourdyn A. Lawrence, and Brigette A. Davis. "Racism and Health: Evidence and Needed Research." *Annual Review of Public Health* 40 (2019): 105–25.

Wool, Zoë. "Mourning, Affect, Sociality: On the Possibilities of Open Grief." *Cultural Anthropology* 35, no. 1 (2020): 40–47.

Woolf, Virginia. *On Being Ill*. 1930. Ashfield, MA: Paris Press, 2002.

Woolf, Virginia. *The Waves*. 1931. Oxford: Oxford University Press, 1992.

www.ingramcontent.com/pod-product-compliance
Lightning Source LLC
Chambersburg PA
CBHW071739270326
41928CB00013B/2735